ULTRASOUND MARKERS FOR FETAL CHROMOSOMAL DEFECTS

FRONTIERS IN FETAL MEDICINE SERIES

SERIES EDITOR: K.H. NICOLAIDES

ULTRASOUND MARKERS FOR FETAL CHROMOSOMAL DEFECTS

R.J.M. SNIJDERS AND K.H. NICOLAIDES

Harris Birthright Research Centre for Fetal Medicine
King's College Hospital Medical School
London, UK

The Parthenon Publishing Group

International Publishers in Medicine, Science & Technology

NEW YORK   LONDON

British Library Cataloguing in Publication Data
Snijders, R.J.M.
   Ultrasound Markers for Fetal Chromosomal Defects – (Frontiers in Fetal Medicine Series)
   I. Title II. Nicolaides, Kypros H.
   III. Series
   618.32042

ISBN 1-85070-610-7

Library of Congress Cataloging-in-Publication Data
Snijders, R.J.M.
Ultrasound markers for fetal chromosomal defects / R.J.M. Snijders and K.H. Nicolaides
   p. cm. – (Frontiers in fetal medicine series)
Includes bibliographical references and index.
ISBN 1-85070-610-7
1. Human chromosome defects–Diagnosis. 2. Fetus–Ultrasonic imaging. 3. Fetus–Defects. 4. Prenatal diagnosis.
I. Nicolaides, K.H. II. Title. III. Series.
[DNLM. 1. Chromosome defects ultrasonography. 2. Ultrasonography, Prenatal. QS 677 S672u 1995]
RG628.3.U68S65 1995
618.3'207543–dc20
DNLM/DLC
for Library of Congress
                95-19473
                CIP

Published in the UK and Europe by
The Parthenon Publishing Group Ltd.
Casterton Hall, Carnforth
Lancs. LA6 2LA, UK

Published in North America by
The Parthenon Publishing Group Inc
One Blue Hill Plaza
Pearl River
New York 10965, USA

Copyright © 1996 Professor K.H. Nicolaides

First published 1996

Composed by AMA Graphics Ltd.

Printed and bound by Bookcraft (Bath) Ltd., Midsomer Norton, UK

Contents

Fetal abnormalities

OVERVIEW

Most fetuses with major chromosomal defects have either external or internal abnormalities which can be recognised by detailed ultrasonographic examination.

This chapter reviews the various published series on the incidence of chromosomal defects for a wide range of anatomical and biometrical abnormalities detected by ultrasound examination during the second and third trimesters of pregnancy.

The studies were mostly from referral centres and therefore the patients examined were preselected. Furthermore, no data were provided on the background risk for chromosomal defects in these populations. Consequently, no conclusions can be drawn as to the true incidence of chromosomal defects for a given fetal abnormality in the general population.

Despite these limitations, the data are useful because they draw attention to the types of chromosomal defects that can be expected with any given abnormality or group of abnormalities. Detection of an abnormality during ultrasound examination should stimulate the search for the other features of the most commonly associated chromosomal defects.

PHENOTYPIC EXPRESSION OF CHROMOSOMAL DEFECTS

In the first trimester, a common feature of many chromosomal defects is increased nuchal translucency thickness (see Chapter 3). In later pregnancy each chromosomal defect has its own syndromal pattern of abnormalities.

Trisomy 21

Trisomy 21 is associated with a tendency for brachycephaly, mild ventriculomegaly, flattening of the face, nuchal oedema (Figure 1.1), atrioventricular septal defects, duodenal atresia and echogenic bowel, mild hydronephrosis, shortening of the limbs, sandal gap and clinodactyly or mid-phalanx hypoplasia of the fifth finger.

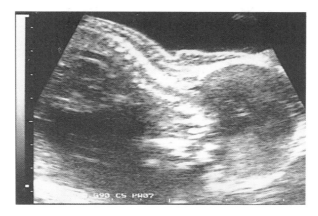

Figure 1.1 Nuchal oedema in a 20 week fetus with trisomy 21.

Trisomy 18

Trisomy 18 is associated with strawberry-shaped head, choroid plexus cysts, absent corpus callosum, enlarged cisterna magna, facial cleft, micrognathia, nuchal oedema, heart defects, diaphragmatic hernia, oesophageal atresia, exomphalos (Figure 1.2), renal defects, myelomeningocoele, growth retardation and shortening of the limbs, radial aplasia, overlapping fingers and talipes or rocker-bottom feet.

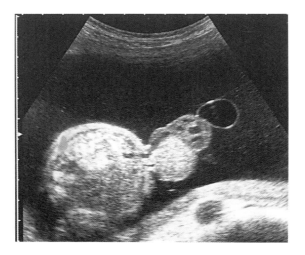

Figure 1.2 Polyhydramnios, hyperechogenic bowel, exomphalos, oedematous umbilical cord and a cord cyst in a 23 week fetus with trisomy 18.

Trisomy 13

In trisomy 13 common defects include holoprosencephaly and associated facial abnormalities (Figure 1.3), microcephaly, cardiac and renal abnormalities (often enlarged and echogenic kidneys), exomphalos and post axial polydactyly.

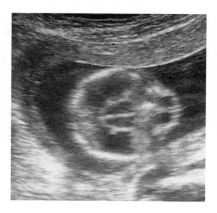

Figure 1.3 Transverse section of the fetal head at the level of the orbits demonstrating severe hypotelorism in a 20 week fetus with holoprosencephaly and trisomy 13.

Triploidy

Triploidy where the extra set of chromosomes is paternally derived is associated with a molar placenta and the pregnancy rarely persists beyond 20 weeks (Figure 1.4). When there is a double maternal chromosome contribution, the pregnancy may persist into the third trimester. The placenta is of normal consistency and the fetus demonstrates severe asymmetrical growth retardation (Figure 1.4). Commonly there is mild ventriculomegaly, micrognathia, cardiac abnormalities, myelomeningocoele, syndactyly, and 'hitch-hiker' toe deformity.

Turner syndrome

The lethal type of Turner syndrome presents with large nuchal cystic hygromata (Figure 1.5), generalised oedema, mild pleural effusions and ascites, cardiac abnormalities and horseshoe kidney (suspected by the ultrasonographic appearance of bilateral mild hydronephrosis).

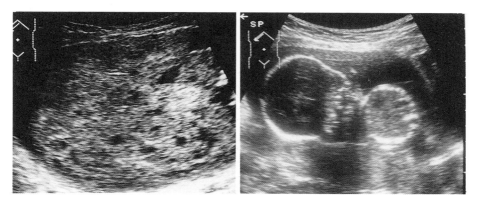

Figure 1.4 The two different phenotypic expressions of triploidy: molar placenta (left) and severe asymmetrical growth retardation (right).

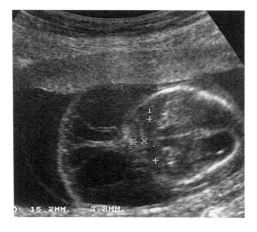

Figure 1.5 Suboccipitobregmatic view of the head demonstrating cystic hygromata in a 16 week fetus with Turner syndrome.

Incidence of abnormalities in common chromosomal defects

The incidence of various abnormalities detected by ultrasound examination during the second and third trimesters of pregnancy, in fetuses with trisomies 21, 18, 13, triploidy and Turner syndrome is shown in Table 1.1. For example, in trisomy 21 the most commonly found abnormalities are nuchal oedema, mild hydronephrosis, relative shortening of the femur and cardiac abnormality.

Table 1.1 Incidence of ultrasound abnormalities in 461 fetuses with chromosomal defects that were examined at the Harris Birthright Research Centre for Fetal Medicine.

| | Chromosomal defect | | | | |
| | Trisomy | | | Triploidy | Turner |
Fetal abnormality	21 n=155	18 n=137	13 n=54	n=50	n=65
Skull/brain					
Strawberry-shaped head	-	54%	-	-	-
Brachycephaly	15%	29%	26%	10%	32%
Microcephaly	-	1%	24%	-	5%
Ventriculomegaly	16%	14%	9%	18%	2%
Holoprosencephaly	-	3%	39%	-	-
Choroid plexus cysts	8%	47%	2%	-	-
Absent corpus callosum	-	7%	-	-	-
Posterior fossa cyst	1%	10%	15%	6%	-
Enlarged cisterna magna	7%	16%	25%	-	-
Face/neck					
Facial cleft	1%	10%	39%	2%	-
Micrognathia	1%	53%	9%	44%	-
Nuchal oedema	38%	5%	22%	4%	6%
Cystic hygromata	1%	2%	-	-	88%
Chest					
Diaphragmatic hernia	-	10%	6%	2%	-
Cardiac abnormality	26%	52%	43%	16%	48%
Abdomen					
Exomphalos	-	31%	17%	2%	-
Duodenal atresia	8%	-	2%	-	-
Absent stomach	3%	20%	2%	2%	-
Mild hydronephrosis	30%	16%	37%	4%	8%
Other renal abnormalities	7%	12%	24%	6%	6%
Other					
Hydrops	20%	4%	7%	2%	80%
Small for gestational age	20%	74%	61%	100%	55%
Relatively short femur	28%	25%	9%	60%	59%
Abnormal hands / feet	25%	72%	52%	76%	2%
Talipes	3%	30%	11%	8%	-

CHROMOSOMAL DEFECTS IN FETAL ABNORMALITIES

Brain abnormalities

Ventriculomegaly

Ventriculomegaly, with a prevalence of 5–25 per 10,000 births, may result from chromosomal and genetic defects, intrauterine haemorrhage or infection but in many cases no clear-cut aetiology is identified. Prenatal diagnosis by ultrasonography is based on the demonstration of dilated lateral cerebral ventricles (Figure 1.6), defined by a ventricle to hemisphere ratio above the 97.5th centile of the normal range for gestation.

In 14 published series on fetal ventriculomegaly the mean prevalence of chromosomal defects was 13%; the prevalence was 2% for fetuses with no other detectable abnormalities and 17% for those with additional abnormalities (Table 1.2). The commonest chromosomal defects were trisomies 21, 18, 13 and triploidy.

Although ventriculomegaly is common in trisomic and triploid fetuses, the majority of fetuses with these chromosomal defects do not have ventriculomegaly (Table 1.1, Figure 1.7).

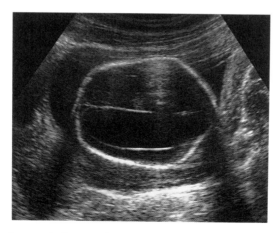

Figure 1.6 Lateral ventriculomegaly and a lemon-shaped head in a fetus with spina bifida.

Table 1.2 Reports on antenatally diagnosed ventriculomegaly providing data on gestational age at diagnosis (GA in weeks) and the prevalence of chromosomal defects in the total group and in the subgroups with isolated ventriculomegaly and those with additional abnormalities. 21 = trisomy 21, 18 = trisomy 18, 13 = trisomy 13, Tripl. = triploidy, Oth = other chromosomal defects.

Author	N	GA	Chromosomal defects							
			Total	Isolated	Multiple	21	18	13	Tripl	Oth
Cochrane *et al* 85	41	18-43	2%	0/9	1/32	-	1	-	-	-
Chervenak *et al* 85a	53	-	8%	?/9	?/44	1	1	-	-	2
Pilu *et al* 86	30	-	10%	?	?	1	2	-	-	-
Nyberg *et al* 87a	31	-	26%	?	?	?	?	?	?	?
Vintzileos *et al* 87	20	18-37	10%	0/6	2/14	-	1	1	-	-
Hudgins *et al* 88	47	>13	2%	0/12	1/35	-	-	-	-	1
Drugan *et al* 89	19	-	26%	?	?	-	1	1	-	2
Rizzo *et al* 90	45	-	11%	0/28	5/17	-	1	1	1	2
Bromley *et al* 91	43	16-37	12%	0/26	5/17	3	1	-	-	1
Anhoury *et al* 91	33	27-31	18%	1/8	5/25	-	2	2	1	1
Brumfield *et al* 91a	24	-	13%	?	?	?	?	?	?	?
Nicolaides *et al* 92e	186	16-38	23%	2/42	40/144	7	12	3	12	5
Holzgreve *et al* 93	118	-	3%	0/28	6/90	1	1	2	-	-
Total	**690**	**13-43**	**13%**	**2%**	**17%**	**13**	**23**	**10**	**14**	**14**

In hydrocephalic fetuses with a chromosomal defect the degree of ventriculomegaly is mild rather than severe (Figure 1.7). Thus, in 420 fetuses with ventriculomegaly diagnosed at the Harris Birthright Research Centre for Fetal Medicine, the overall frequency of chromosomal defects was 19%; in those with a ventricle to hemisphere ratio of 2–6 standard deviations above the normal mean for gestation, the frequency was 22%, whereas in those with more severe ventriculomegaly the frequency was only 6% (Table 1.3).

Table 1.3 Prevalence of chromosomal defects in 420 fetuses with ventriculomegaly in relation to the degree of deviation from the normal mean for gestation and the absence (isolated) or presence (multiple) of other abnormalities.

Ventricle/hemisphere (SDs above normal mean)	Total	Isolated	Multiple
2.0-3.9	22%	1/45 (2%)	52/196 (27%)
4.0-5.9	21%	3/35 (9%)	17/ 62 (27%)
6.0-7.9	8%	1/16 (6%)	3/ 37 (8%)
≥8.0	3%	0/10 (0%)	1/ 19 (5%)

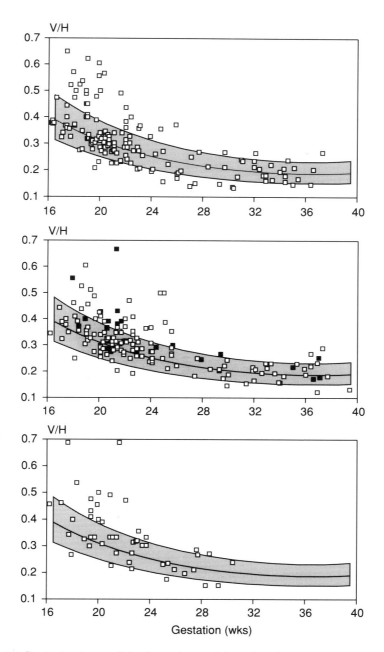

Figure 1.7 Posterior horn of the lateral ventricle to hemisphere ratio (V/H) in 155 fetuses with trisomy 21 (top), 137 with trisomy 18 (□, middle) and 54 with trisomy 13 (■, middle) and 50 with triploidy (bottom) diagnosed at the Harris Birthright Research Centre for Fetal Medicine plotted on the normal range for gestation (mean, 97.5th and 2.5th centiles).

Holoprosencephaly

Holoprosencephaly has an incidence of approximately 1 per 10,000 births, but may affect as many as 0.4% of all conceptuses (Matsunaga *et al* 1977). It encompasses a heterogeneous group of cerebral malformations resulting from either failure or incomplete cleavage of the forebrain. Although in many cases the cause is a chromosomal defect or a genetic disorder with an autosomal dominant or recessive mode of transmission, in the majority of cases the aetiology is unknown. Prenatal diagnosis by ultrasonography is based on the demonstration of a single dilated midline ventricle replacing the two lateral ventricles (Figure 1.8).

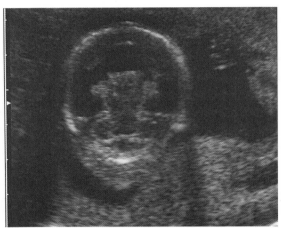

Figure 1.8 Holoprosencephaly in a 20 week fetus with trisomy 13. Note the single ventricle but a normal midbrain and cerebellum.

In the published studies on fetal holoprosencephaly, the mean prevalence of chromosomal defects was 33%; the prevalence was 4% for fetuses with apparently isolated holoprosencephaly and 39% for those with additional abnormalities (Table 1.4).

The commonest chromosomal defects were trisomies 13 and 18. However, the majority of fetuses with these chromosomal defects do not have holoprosencephaly (Table 1.1).

Fetal holoprosencephaly is commonly associated with a wide variety of mid-facial abnormalities. Berry *et al* (1990) examined

Table 1.4 Reports on antenatally diagnosed holoprosencephaly providing data on gestational age at diagnosis (GA in weeks) and the frequency of chromosomal defects in the total group and in the subgroups with isolated holoprosencephaly and those with additional abnormalities. 18 = trisomy 18, 13 = trisomy 13.

Author	N	GA	Chromosomal defects					
			Total	Isolated	Multiple	18	13	Other
Filly *et al* 84	5	23-30	20%	0/1	1/4	-	-	1
Chervenak *et al* 85b	7	27-37	57%	-	4/7	-	2	2
Nyberg *et al* 87b	11	14-38	55%	1/3	5/8	-	4	2
Berry *et al* 90*	38	>26	29%	0/12	11/26	2	8	1
Hsieh *et al* 92	10	17-36	50%	-	5/10	2	3	-
Nicolaides *et al* 92e	58	-	26%	0/7	15/51	3	11	1
Wilson *et al* 92	3	-	67%	-	2/3	-	2	-
Total	**132**	**14-38**	**33%**	**4%**	**39%**	**7**	**30**	**7**

*Cases are included in Nicolaides *et al* 92e.

whether the frequency of chromosomal defects is increased even when the only additional abnormalities are facial. They reported chromosomal defects in 46% of fetuses with holoprosencephaly and extrafacial defects but in none of the fetuses where the holoprosencephaly was either isolated or associated with facial abnormalities only.

Microcephaly

Microcephaly, with an incidence of about 1 per 1,000 births, may be the consequence of chromosomal defects, genetic syndromes, haemorrhage, infection, teratogens and radiation.

Prenatal diagnosis is based on the identification of a disproportionally reduced head circumference and the associated intracranial pathology. However, the intracranial anatomy may be normal, in which case the condition is defined by a biparietal diameter below the 1st centile or by a head circumference to femur length ratio below the 2.5th centile of the normal range for gestation. In milder cases, diagnosis requires the demonstration of a progressive decrease in the head circumference until it falls below the 5th centile, in the presence of normal growth of the abdomen and femur. This may not become apparent before 26 weeks of gestation.

In a series of 2,086 fetuses that were karyotyped because of fetal malformations or growth retardation, the diagnosis of micro-cephaly was made if the head circumference was below the 5th centile and the head circumference to femur length ratio was below the 2.5th centile (Nicolaides *et al* 1992e). There were 52 cases of microcephaly and eight (15%) of these had chromosomal defects. Eydoux *et al* (1989) reported chromosomal defects in five (25%) of 20 cases. In the combined data from these two series, 12 of the 13 chromosomally abnormal fetuses had additional abnormalities and the commonest chromosomal defect was trisomy 13. However, it should be noted that the majority of fetuses with trisomy 13 do not have microcephaly and those that do usually have holoprosencephaly (Figure 1.9).

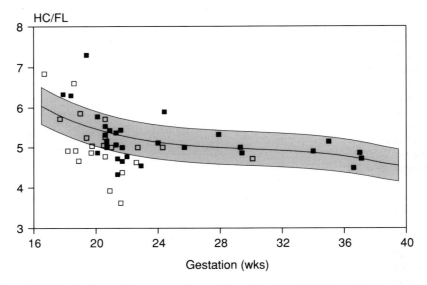

Figure 1.9 Head circumference to femur length ratio (HC/FL) in 54 fetuses with trisomy 13, with (■) or without (□) holoprosencephaly, diagnosed at the Harris Birthright Research Centre for Fetal Medicine plotted on the normal range for gestation (mean, 95th and 5th centiles).

Choroid plexus cysts

Choroid plexus cysts (Figure 1.10) are found in approximately 1% of fetuses at 16–24 weeks of gestation but in more than 90% of cases they resolve by 26–28 weeks and are of no pathological significance. Several reports have documented an association between choroid plexus cysts and chromosomal defects, particularly trisomy 18 (Table 1.5). The mean prevalence of chromosomal defects in the various published series was 8%, with an 1% prevalence for apparently isolated lesions and 46% for those with additional abnormalities.

Table 1.5 Reports on antenatally diagnosed choroid plexus cysts providing data on gestational age at diagnosis (GA in weeks) and the prevalence of chromosomal defects in the total group and in the subgroups with isolated choroid plexus cysts and those with additional abnormalities. 21 = trisomy 21, 18 = trisomy 18, Oth = other chromosomal defects

Author	N	GA	Chromosomal defects					
			Total	Isolated	Multiple	21	18	Oth
Nicolaides *et al* 86	4	18-24	75%	0/0	3/4	-	3	-
Ricketts *et al* 87	4	19-23	25%	0/3	1/1	1	-	-
Chitkara *et al* 88	41	16-33	2%	0/37	1/4	-	1	-
Clark *et al* 88	5	16-22	0%	0/5	-	-	-	-
DeRoo *et al* 88	16	14-21	0%	0/16	-	-	-	-
Benacerraf *et al* 89	38	15-28	0%	0/38	-	-	-	-
Chan *et al* 89	13	15-24	0%	0/13	-	-	-	-
Hertzberg *et al* 89	31	>13	0%	0/29	0/2	-	-	-
Gabrielli *et al* 89	82	16-28	5%	0/77	4/5	-	4	-
Ostlere *et al* 90	100	16-18	3%	0/91	3/9	-	3	-
Thorpe-Beeston 90*	78	15-37	26%	0/44	20/34	2	16	2
Achiron *et al* 91	30	19-21	17%	1/29	1/1	-	5	-
Chinn *et al* 91	38	15-24	2%	0/36	1/2	-	-	1
Platt *et al* 91	62	15-22	6%	0/58	4/4	1	3	-
Twining *et al* 91b	19	18-20	11%	0/16	2/3	1	1	-
Zerres *et al* 92	25	?	20%	0/14	5/11	1	4	-
Nadel *et al* 92	234	14-27	5%	0/220	12/14	-	11	1
Perpignano *et al* 92	83	14-33	7%	5/82	1/1	1	4	1
Howard *et al* 92	51	18-20	2%	1/49	0/2	-	1	-
Nicolaides *et al* 92e	121	16-38	28%	1/49	33/72	2	30	2
Rebaud *et al* 92	29	18-36	7%	0/26	2/3	1	1	-
Wilson *et al* 92	8	?	13%	0/6	1/2	-	1	-
Oettinger *et al* 93	14	?	14%	0/12	2/2	1	1	-
Porto *et al* 93	63	15-22	10%	2/59	4/4	2	3	1
Nava *et al* 94	211	16-23	4%	4/193	4/18	2	4	2
Snijders *et al* 94	332	16-23	12%	2/234	43/98	4	38	3
Walkinshaw *et al* 94	152	17-19	33%	4/140	0/12	1	3	-
Total	**1806**	**14-38**	**8%**	**1%**	**46%**	**18**	**121**	**11**

* Cases are included in Nicolaides *et al* 92e

Snijders *et al* (1994) have suggested that, since the frequency of chromosomal defects is associated with maternal age, it is possible that the wide range in the reported prevalence of chromosomal defects is the mere consequence of differences in the maternal age distribution of the populations examined in the various studies. If the choroid plexus cysts are apparently isolated, then the maternal age-related risk for trisomy 18 is only marginally increased. A method of evaluating chromosomal markers in relation to maternal age is proposed in Chapter 2.

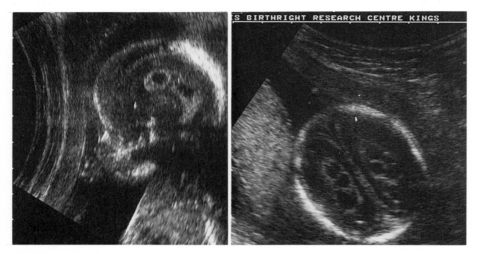

Figure 1.10 Bilateral, multiple choroid plexus cysts in a 20 week fetus with trisomy 18.

Absent corpus callosum

Agenesis of the corpus callosum may be an isolated finding of no pathological significance, but it is also found in association with genetic syndromes and chromosomal defects (Vergani *et al* 1994).

Three studies on a total of 17 fetuses with absent corpus callosum reported trisomy 13 in one fetus who had additional abnormalities (Comstock *et al* 1985, Lockwood *et al* 1988, Vergani *et al* 1994). We diagnosed absence of the corpus callosum in 7% of 137 fetuses with trisomy 18 (Table 1.1) but never as an isolated abnormality.

Short frontal lobe

Trisomy 21 is associated with brachycephaly, which is thought to be due to reduced growth of the frontal lobe. Frontothalamic distance is measured from the inner table of the frontal bone to the posterior thalamus. Bahado-Singh *et al* (1992) reported that in 19 trisomy 21 fetuses at 16–21 weeks of gestation, the frontothalamic distance to biparietal diameter ratio was significantly lower than in 125 normal controls; in 21% of fetuses with trisomy 21 the ratio was below the 5th centile. These findings await confirmation from further studies.

Posterior fossa abnormalities

The Dandy–Walker malformation (cystic dilatation in the area of the cisterna magna, with partial or complete agenesis of the vermis) may occur as part of Mendelian disorders, such as Meckel syndrome or a chromosomal defect, but in most cases the aetiology is unknown (Figure 1.11).

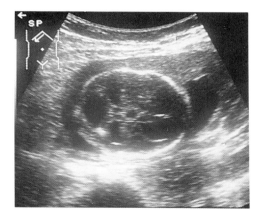

Figure 1.11 Posterior fossa cyst in an 18 week fetus with trisomy 18.

In the combined data from five series on a total of 101 fetuses with enlarged posterior fossa, the mean frequency of associated chromosomal defects, mainly trisomy 18, was 44% (Table 1.6).

Table 1.6 Reports on antenatally diagnosed posterior fossa cyst providing data on gestational age at diagnosis (GA in weeks) and the frequency of chromosomal defects in the total group and in the subgroups with isolated cysts and those with additional abnormalities. 18 = trisomy 18, 13 = trisomy 13.

Author	N	GA	Chromosomal defects					
			Total	Isolated	Multiple	18	13	Other
Nyberg *et al* 91	33	18-38	55%	0/5	18/28	12	3	2
Wilson *et al* 92	2	?	0%	0/1	0/1	-	-	-
Watson *et al* 92	4	14-21	0%	?	?	-	-	-
Estroff *et al* 92	17	17-38	30%	0/6	5/11	2	1	2
Nicolaides *et al* 92e	45	16-38	47%	0/1	21/44	8	6	4
Total	**101**	**14-38**	**44%**	**0%**	**52%**	**22**	**10**	**8**

The normal range of cisterna magna diameter with gestation and the values from 113 fetuses with trisomies 21, 18 or 13 diagnosed at the Harris Birthright Research Centre for Fetal Medicine are shown in Figure 1.12.

The diameter was above the 95th centile in 7%, 16% and 25% of the fetuses with trisomies 21, 18 and 13 respectively.

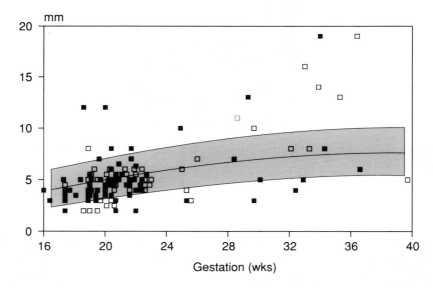

Figure 1.12 Cisterna magna diameter in 54 fetuses with trisomy 21 (□) and 59 with trisomies 18 or 13 (■) diagnosed at the Harris Birthright Centre for Fetal Medicine plotted on the normal range for gestation (mean, 95th and 5th centiles).

Abnormal shape of the head

Strawberry-shaped skull

In some fetuses with trisomy 18 there is a characteristic shape of the head that is best seen in the suboccipitobregmatic view (Figure 1.13). There is flattening of the occiput and narrowing of the frontal part of the head. The most likely explanation for the narrow frontal region is hypoplasia of the face and frontal cerebral lobes. Similarly, flattening of the occiput may be due to hypoplasia of the hindbrain. In a series of 54 fetuses with strawberry-shaped head, they all had additional malformations and 44 (81%) had chromosomal defects (Nicolaides *et al* 1992c). Strawberry-shaped skull is a 'gestalt' marker, rather than a measurable feature. The extent to which the introduction of techniques such as pattern recognition analysis will provide more objective description of the marker remains to be determined.

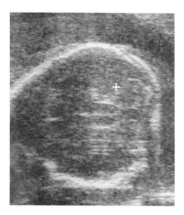

Figure 1.13 Strawberry-shaped head in a fetus with trisomy 18 diagnosed at 22 weeks of gestation.

Brachycephaly

Brachycephaly is characterised by relative shortening of the occipitofrontal diameter. It is found in association with chromosomal defects and genetic syndromes, such as Roberts syndrome. In postnatal life it is well recognised that children with Down syndrome have brachycephaly. However, two prenatal ultrasonographic studies have found no difference in the mean cephalic index (biparietal to occipitofrontal diameter ratio) between 25 second-trimester fetuses with trisomy 21 and 325 normal controls (Perry *et al* 1984, Shah *et al* 1990b). In our series of 451 fetuses with chromosomal defects, the mean cephalic index was increased but in the majority of cases the index was below the 97.5th centile; brachycephaly was observed in 15% of fetuses with trisomy 21, 28% of those with trisomies 18 or 13, 10% of those with triploidy and 32% of those with Turner syndrome (Figure 1.14).

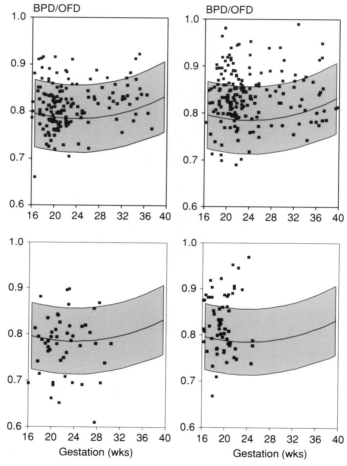

Figure 1.14 Biparietal to occipitofrontal diameter (BPD/OFD) in 155 fetuses with trisomy 21 (top, left), 137 with trisomy 18 and 54 with trisomy 13 (top, right), 50 with triploidy (bottom, left) and 65 with Turner syndrome (bottom, right) diagnosed at the Harris Birthright Research Centre for Fetal Medicine plotted on the normal range for gestation (mean, 97.5th and 2.5th centiles).

Facial abnormalities

Facial cleft and other facial abnormalities are common features of certain chromosomal defects. These abnormalities are usually detected by careful examination of the face after the diagnosis of other fetal abnormalities and/or growth retardation.

Facial cleft

Cleft lip and/or palate (Figure 1.15) are among the commonest congenital abnormalities, found in approximately 1 per 700 live births, and both genetic and environmental factors are implicated in their causation.

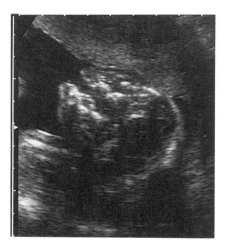

Figure 1.15 Transverse section at the level of the upper lip demonstrating a facial cleft in an 18 week fetus with trisomy 13.

Postnatally, chromosomal defects are found in less than 1% of babies with facial cleft (Pashayan *et al* 1983). However, in seven prenatal series reporting on a total of 118 fetuses, 40% had chromosomal defects, most commonly trisomies 13 and 18; in all fetuses with chromosomal defects there were additional abnormalities (Table 1.7).

In our centre a facial cleft was diagnosed in 10% of fetuses with trisomy 18 and in 39% of those with trisomy 13 (Table 1.1).

Table 1.7 Reports on antenatally diagnosed facial cleft providing data on gestational age at diagnosis (GA in weeks) and the frequency of chromosomal defects in the total group and in the subgroups with isolated facial cleft and those with additional abnormalities. 18 = trisomy 18, 13 = trisomy 13.

Author	N	GA	Chromosomal defects					
			Total	Isolated	Multiple	18	13	Other
Saltzman *et al* 86	12	18-37	33%	0/2	4/10	1	3	-
Hsieh *et al* 91	6	28-37	50%	-	3/6	2	1	-
Wilson *et al* 92	3	?	0%	0/2	0/1	-	-	-
Benacerraf *et al* 93	22	15-40	27%	0/9	6/13	1	5	-
Nicolaides *et al* 93	64	17-37	48%	0/8	31/56	10	15	6
Turner & Twining 93	7	18-32	29%	0/2	2/5	1	1	-
Bronshtein *et al* 94	4	15	25%	0/3	1/1	1	-	-
Total	**118**	**15-40**	**40%**	**0%**	**51%**	**16**	**25**	**6**

The high prevalence of chromosomal defects and other abnormalities in the prenatal studies indicates that the populations examined were preselected. Presumably, in the majority of cases detailed ultrasound examination leading to the diagnosis of facial clefting was performed in referral centres because routine scanning had demonstrated the presence of a variety of extrafacial defects. This is discussed further in Chapter 2.

Micrognathia

Micrognathia (Figure 1.16) is a non-specific finding in a wide range of genetic syndromes and chromosomal defects. In two studies reporting on 65 cases where micrognathia was diagnosed antenatally, all fetuses had additional malformations and/or growth retardation. The prevalence of chromosomal defects was 62% and the commonest was trisomy 18 (Nicolaides *et al* 1993, Turner & Twining 1993).

Conversely, we diagnosed micrognathia in 53% of fetuses with trisomy 18 and 44% of those with triploidy, while postmortem studies have demonstrated micrognathia to be present in more than 80% of these fetuses (Benacerraf *et al* 1986a). This suggests that at present only severe micrognathia is amenable to prenatal diagnosis.

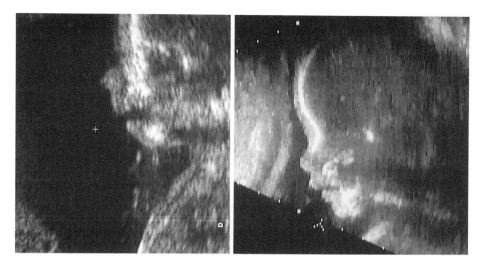

Figure 1.16 Micrognathia in an 18 week fetus with trisomy 18 (left) and a normal profile (right).

Ocular and nasal abnormalities

Eye abnormalities, such as hypotelorism and cyclopia, and nasal defects, such as nasal aplasia or hypoplasia, single nostril, or proboscis (Figure 1.17) are often seen in the presence of holoprosencephaly, and they are associated with trisomies 13 and 18 (Nicolaides *et al* 1993).

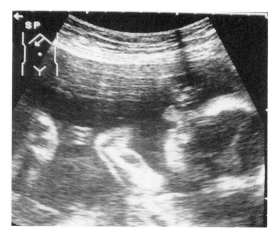

Figure 1.17 Profile of a 19 week fetus with trisomy 13 demonstrating proboscis.

Although all chromosomally abnormal fetuses with holoprosencephaly have extra-craniofacial abnormalities, the risk for chromosomal defects increases if facial defects are also present (Berry *et al* 1990).

Macroglossia

Postnatally, macroglossia and a flat profile are common features of trisomy 21. Antenatally these abnormalities are rarely diagnosed unless other features of trisomy 21 are found. In a series of 69 fetuses with trisomy 21, macroglossia was diagnosed in 10% of those examined at <28 weeks and 20% of those diagnosed at >28 weeks (Nicolaides *et al* 1993). It is possible that with advancing gestation there is progressive enlargement and/or protrusion of the tongue to account for the higher prevalence of macroglossia at term.

Small ears

Chromosomally abnormal infants often have small ears. Indeed, an anthropomorphic study of Down syndrome babies noted that a decrease in ear length is the most striking deviation of all measurements (Thelander & Pryor 1966). Aase *et al* (1973) reported that the ear length was below the third centile in 23 of 25 neonates with Down syndrome. Three prenatal ultrasonographic studies have confirmed that the ear length of fetuses with chromosomal defects is decreased (Birnholz & Farrell 1988, Lettieri *et al* 1993, Awwad *et al* 1994).

Neck abnormalities

Nuchal cystic hygromata

Nuchal cystic hygromata are developmental abnormalities of the lymphatic system. Although they are rarely seen postnatally, they are found in 0.5% of spontaneously aborted fetuses (Byrne *et al* 1984). Prenatal diagnosis by ultrasonography is based on the demonstration of a bilateral, septated, cystic structure, located in the occipitocervical region. This condition should be distinguished from nuchal oedema, which has a high association with trisomies, or unilateral cervical cysts, which are usually detected in the third trimester and have a good prognosis after postnatal surgery.

Reports on antenatally diagnosed cystic hygromata have established an association with hydrops fetalis, found in 40–100% of the cases, congenital heart defects, in 0–92% of the cases, and chromosomal defects in 46–90% of the fetuses, the commonest being Turner syndrome (Table 1.8).

Table 1.8 Reports on antenatally diagnosed cystic hygromata providing data on gestational age at diagnosis (GA in weeks) and the frequency of chromosomal defects in the total group and in the subgroups with isolated cystic hygromata and those with additional abnormalities. 21 = trisomy 21, 18 = trisomy 18, Oth = other chromosomal defects.

Author	N	GA	Chromosomal defects						
			Total	Isolated	Multiple	21	18	45X	Oth
Chervenak et al 83	15	18-29	73%	?	?	-	-	11	-
Newman et al 84	3	16-26	67%	- / -	2/3	1	-	1	-
Redford et al 84	5	17-26	80%	- / -	4/5	1	1	2	-
Marchese et al 85	6	16-20	83%	- / -	5/6	-	1	4	-
Pearce et al 85	22	16-26	77%	?	?	2	1	14	-
Nicolaides et al 85	8	16-29	75%	- / -	6/8	1	-	5	-
Carr et al 86	5	17-28	60%	- / -	3/5	1	-	2	-
Palmer et al 87	8	16-28	75%	?	?	1	-	4	1
Hegge et al 88	4	15-17	75%	0/1	3/3	1	-	2	-
Abramowicz et al 89	16	15-31	63%	?	?	3	1	6	-
Miyabara et al 89	8	18-23	88%	1/1	6/7	2	-	3	2
Holzgreve et al 90	15	?	67%	?	?	2	1	7	-
Rizzo et al 90	13	15-27	77%	10/12	0/1	1	1	8	-
Tanniradorn et al 90	11	16-23	64%	?	?	-	1	5	1
Azar et al 91*	44	16-25	75%	2/3	31/41	1	1	31	-
MacLeod et al 91	15	16-38	67%	0/2	10/13	3	2	3	2
Brumfield et al 91a	11	?	73%	?	?	?	?	?	?
Bernard et al 91	20	15-28	65%	1/2	12/18	5	1	12	4
Nicolaides et al 92e	52	16-35	67%	0/4	35/48	1	1	33	-
Wilson et al 92	9	?	11%	1/4	0/5	-	-	-	1
Gagnon et al 92	9	?	78%	?	?	1	1	5	-
Hsieh et al 92	15	?	47%	?	?	-	-	7	-
Ville et al 92	6	16-26	67%	0/0	4/6	-	1	3	-
Total	276	15-38	68%	52%	71%	26	13	163	11

* Cases are included in Nicolaides et al 1992e

Azar et al (1991) suggested that the wide range in the reported prevalence of hydrops fetalis, cardiac defects and both the presence and types of chromosomal defects may be a consequence of differences in the diagnostic criteria for cystic hygromata used in the various reports. In their study, which examined only fetuses with septated, cervical, dorsal hygromata, 75% had chromosomal defects; Turner syndrome accounted for 94%. In a fetus with cystic hygromata the risk for Turner syndrome is increased if the mother is young, if there is a fetal cardiac defect and if the head circumference to femur length ratio is increased. Unlike with most other abnormalities, in cystic hygromata, the prevalence of chromosomal defects is high, even for apparently isolated hygromata. The two most likely explanations for this finding are first, the total number of reported cases is small and second, the most common chromosomal defect is Turner syndrome, where the associated coarctation of the aorta can be difficult to diagnose antenatally.

Although chromosomally abnormal fetuses are often growth retarded, in fetuses with cystic hygromata, measurement of the abdominal circumference is not a useful predictor of karyotype because this measurement is affected by the presence or absence of ascites and generalised oedema. In contrast, measurements of head circumference and femur length are useful because the degree of femur shortening in fetuses with Turner syndrome is greater than in chromosomally normal fetuses (Figure 1.18).

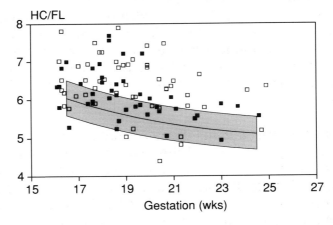

Figure 1.18 Head circumference to femur length ratio (HC/FL) in 99 fetuses with cystic hygromata diagnosed at the Harris Birthright Research Centre for Fetal Medicine plotted on the normal range for gestation (mean, 95th and 5th centiles). In the 58 fetuses with Turner syndrome (□) the degree of femur shortening is greater than in chromosomally normal fetuses (■).

Nuchal oedema

Benacerraf *et al* (1985, 1987b) noted the association between increased soft tissue thickening on the posterior aspect of the neck and trisomy 21. In a series of 1,704 consecutive amniocenteses at 15–20 weeks' gestation in which there were 11 fetuses with trisomy 21, 45% of the trisomic and 0.06% of the normal fetuses had nuchal thickness more than 5 mm. Similarly, Lynch *et al* (1989), who retrospectively examined the sonograms of nine pairs of discordant twins, found increased nuchal thickening in five of the nine fetuses with trisomy 21 but in none of the normal co-twins. However, Perrella *et al* (1988) retrospectively examined the sonograms of 14 fetuses with trisomy 21 and 128 normal controls and found increased nuchal thickening in only 21% of the trisomic fetuses and in 9% of the normals. Similarly, Nyberg *et al* (1990) reviewed the sonographic findings of 68 consecutive fetuses with trisomy 21 at 14–24 weeks of gestation and found increased nuchal thickening in only five (7%).

A prospective multicentre study of 1,382 women undergoing amniocentesis at 14–20 weeks of gestation investigated the value of nuchal skinfold thickness as a screening test for Down syndrome (Donnenfeld *et al* 1994). There was no statistically significant difference between the chromosomally normal (median = 3.1 mm) and Down syndrome fetuses (median = 3.2 mm). Using a nuchal skinfold thickness of more than 5 mm as a screening test, the detection rate for Down syndrome was 8% and the false positive rate was 1.2%. The authors concluded that this was a poor and unreliable screening test for Down syndrome.

Nicolaides *et al* (1992a) considered nuchal oedema to be present if in the mid-sagittal plane of the neck there was subcutaneous oedema (at least 7 mm) that produced a characteristic tremor on ballottement of the fetal head. This was distinguished from nuchal cystic hygromata and hydrops fetalis, in which there was generalised oedema. In a series of 144 fetuses with nuchal oedema, 37% had chromosomal defects, mainly trisomy 21, but also other trisomies, deletions or translocations, triploidy and Turner syndrome (Nicolaides *et al* 1992e). Furthermore the chromosomally normal fetuses had a very poor prognosis because in many cases there was an underlying skeletal dysplasia, genetic syndrome or cardiac defect. In a total of 371 cases in nine reports on fetal nuchal thickening, 33% had chromosomal defects and the commonest was trisomy 21 (Table 1.9). The most likely explanation for the high prevalence of chromosomal defects even for apparently isolated nuchal oedema is that the most common defect is trisomy 21, where the associated abnormalities are usually subtle.

Table 1.9 Studies on antenatally diagnosed nuchal oedema reporting the prevalence of chromosomal defects in the total group and in the subgroups with isolated oedema and those with additional abnormalities. 21 = trisomy 21, 18 = trisomy 18, Oth = other chromosomal defects, Isol = isolated chromosomal defects

Author	N	GA	Chromosomal defects						
			Total	Isol	Multiple	21	18	45X	Oth
Toi *et al* 87	10	15-20	40%	4/9	0/1	4	-	-	-
Perrella *et al* 88	15	15-21	20%	?	?	3	-	-	-
Crane & Gray 91	47	16-21	26%	5/?	7/?	12	-	-	-
Kirk *et al* 92	30	15-20	40%	6/20	6/10	9	-	-	2
Nicolaides *et al* 92e	144	16-38	37%	0/12	53/132	31	5	3	14
Benacerraf *et al* 92	42	14-21	33%	8/36	6/6	11	-	3	-
DeVore & Alfi 93	23	14-23	39%	0/7	9/16	7	1	-	1
Donnenfeld 94	17	14-20	6%	1/17	- / -	1	-	-	-
Watson *et al* 94	43	14-21	37%	?	?	7	3	4	2
Total	371	14-38	33%	19%	45%	85	9	10	19

Hydrops fetalis

Hydrops fetalis (Figure 1.19), with an incidence of about 1 per 1,000 births, is characterised by generalised skin oedema and pericardial, pleural, or ascitic effusions. Hydrops is a non-specific finding in a wide variety of fetal and maternal disorders, including haematological, chromosomal, cardiovascular, renal, pulmonary, gastrointestinal, hepatic and metabolic abnormalities, congenital infection, neoplasms and malformations of the placenta or umbilical cord. While in many instances the underlying cause may be determined by detailed ultrasound scanning, frequently the abnormality remains unexplained even after expert postmortem examination.

In a review of the literature up to 1989, Jauniaux *et al* (1990) reported chromosomal defects in 16% of 600 fetuses with non-immune hydrops; the commonest abnormalities were trisomy 21 and Turner syndrome, found in 38% and 35% of the cases respectively. In our series of 214 fetuses with non-rhesus hydrops (excluding those with cystic hygromata, mentioned above), 12% had chromosomal defects, mainly trisomy 21 (Nicolaides *et al* 1992e).

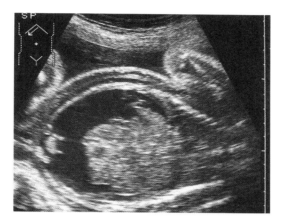

Figure 1.19 Ascites and skin oedema in a 20 week fetus with trisomy 21.

Thoracic abnormalities

Diaphragmatic hernia

Diaphragmatic hernia, with an incidence of about 1 per 3,000 births, can be diagnosed by the ultrasonographic demonstration of stomach, intestines or liver in the thorax and the associated mediastinal shift to the opposite side (Figure 1.20).

Polyhydramnios, ascites and other malformations, predominantly craniospinal and cardiac, are often present. In seven prenatal series reporting on a total of 173 fetuses with diaphragmatic hernia, 18% had chromosomal defects, most commonly trisomy 18; the prevalence was 2% for those with apparently isolated diaphragmatic hernia and 34% for those with multiple additional abnormalities (Table 1.10).

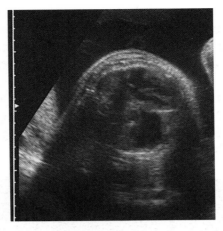

Figure 1.20 Cross-section of the thorax in a 20 week fetus with trisomy 18 demonstrating diaphragmatic hernia.

Table 1.10 Reports on antenatally diagnosed diaphragmatic hernia providing data on gestational age at diagnosis (GA in weeks) and the prevalence of chromosomal defects in the total group and in the subgroups with isolated hernia and those with additional abnormalities. 18 = trisomy 18.

Author	N	GA	Chromosomal defects				
			Total	Isolated	Multiple	18	Other
Benacerraf *et al* 87a	19	15-41	21%	? /10	?/9	2	2
Gagnon *et al* 92	5	14-37	40%	0 / ?	2/?	1	1
Thorpe-Beeston *et al* 89*	36	17-38	31%	0/17	15/19	6	5
Fogel *et al* 91**	10	16-40	40%	2/8	2/2	1	3
Nicolaides *et al* 92e	79	17-38	22%	0/38	17/41	10	7
Wilson *et al* 92	5	?	60%	-	3/5	3	-
Sharland *et al* 92	55	15-38	4%	0/42	2/13	1	1
Total	**173**	**14-41**	**18%**	**2%**	**34%**	**18**	**14**

* Cases are included in Nicolaides *et al* (1992).
** The report only mentioned presence or absence of heart defects.

Cardiac abnormalities

Gross structural abnormalities of the heart or major blood vessels which have, or potentially have, effects on the proper functioning of the heart are found in approximately 1% of live births and 2–10% of stillbirths. While some of the defects resolve spontaneously (e.g. ventricular septal defect) and others are easily correctable, major structural abnormalities are either inoperable or carry high operative risks (e.g. hypoplastic left heart). The occurrence of heart defects probably depends on the interplay of multiple genetic and environmental factors (Nora & Nora 1978).

Echocardiography has been applied successfully to the prenatal assessment of the fetal cardiac function and structure and has led to the prenatal diagnosis of most moderate to major cardiac abnormalities (Figure 1.21).

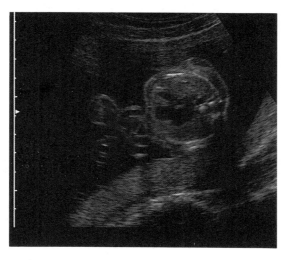

Figure 1.21 Four chamber view of the fetal heart demonstrating an atrio-ventricular septal defect in a 20 week fetus with trisomy 21.

Nora and Nora (1978) reported that heart defects are found in more than 99% of fetuses with trisomy 18, in 90% of those with trisomy 13, 50% of trisomy 21, 40–50% of those with deletions or partial trisomies involving chromosomes 4, 5, 8, 9, 13, 14, 18, or 22 and in 35% of 45,X0.

Prenatal studies of ultrasonographically detectable fetal cardiac abnormalities have reported chromosomal defects in 28% of 829 cases (Table 1.11). The commonest defects were trisomies 21, 18, 13 and Turner syndrome. Chromosomal defects were found in 16% of cases with apparently isolated heart defects and in 65% of those with additional abnormalities. There are two possible explanations for the high frequency of chromosomal defects even for apparently isolated cardiac abnormalities. First, the defect involved is trisomy 21 where associated abnormalities are subtle, and second, the results are mainly due to one study where other abnormalities may have been missed.

Table 1.11 Reports on antenatally diagnosed heart defects providing data on the frequency of chromosomal defects in the total group and in the subgroups with isolated heart defect and those with additional abnormalities. 21 = trisomy 21, 18 = trisomy 18, 13 = trisomy 13, Oth = other chromosomal abnormalities.

Author	N	Chromosomal defects							
		Total	Isolated	Multiple	21	18	13	45X	Oth
Allan *et al* 91	467	16%	13/?	64/?	25	25	6	9	12
Blake *et al* 91	17	18%	0/11	3/6	-	-	1	2	-
Nicolaides *et al* 92e	156	65%	0/4	101/152	21	37	14	16	13
Smythe *et al* 92	158	28%	?	?	16	16	5	3	5
Paladini *et al* 93	31	48%	5/17	10/14	6	4	4	-	1
Total	**829**	**29%**	**16%**	**66%**	**68**	**82**	**30**	**30**	**31**

Recently there has been interest in the clinical significance of echogenic foci or 'golf balls' within the ventricles of the fetal heart (Figure 1.22).

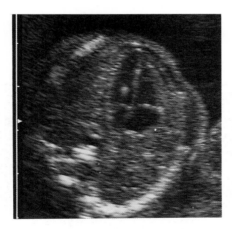

Figure 1.22 Echogenic focus in the left ventricle of the heart in a chromosomally normal 20 week fetus.

The prevalence in routine second trimester scans is 0.5–1.2% and their size varies from 1mm to 6mm (Twining 1993, How *et al* 1994).

Histological studies have shown these foci to be due to mineralisation within a papillary muscle (Brown *et al* 1994). Follow up studies of fetuses with echogenic foci have demonstrated normal ventricular function and competent atrioventricular valves (How *et al* 1994). Although in some cases there is a chromosomal defect, in such fetuses the echogenic foci are associated with multiple other abnormalities (Twining 1993).

Gastrointestinal tract abnormalities

Oesophageal atresia

Oesophageal atresia is a sporadic condition found in 2–10 per 10,000 births and, in 90% of the cases, there is an associated tracheoesophageal fistula. Prenatally the diagnosis of oesophageal atresia is suspected when, in the presence of polyhydramnios, repeated ultrasonographic examinations fail to demonstrate the fetal stomach (Figure 1.23); other possible diagnoses include lack of fetal swallowing, due to arthrogryposis, and intrathoracic compression, due to cystic adenomatoid malformation or pleural effusion. In the presence of a tracheoesophageal fistula, the stomach bubble may be normal.

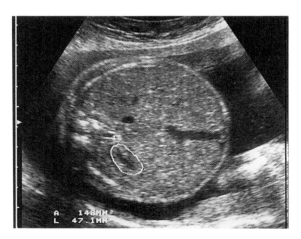

Figure 1.23 Thick walled, collapsed stomach in a fetus with oesophageal atresia.

Postnatally, chromosomal defects were reported in 3–4% of neonates with oesophageal atresia (German *et al* 1976, Louhimo & Lindahl 1983). In a prenatal series of 20 fetuses with no visible stomach and the presumptive diagnosis of oesophageal atresia, 85% had trisomy 18 and in all cases there were additional abnormalities (Nicolaides *et al* 1992d). The most likely explanation for the very high frequency of chromosomal defects found prenatally, compared to that after birth, is that trisomy 18 fetuses often die *in utero* or they are born at previable gestations due to the polyhydramnios; unlike chromosomally normal fetuses, in trisomy 18 oesophageal atresia is not usually associated with tracheoesophageal fistula. In addition, as with facial defects, in the majority of fetuses with oesophageal atresia the diagnosis was made by detailed ultrasound examination after the detection of other abnormalities or growth retardation at routine scanning.

Duodenal atresia

Duodenal atresia or stenosis has an incidence of 1 in 10,000 live births. In most cases the condition is sporadic, although a familial inheritance has been suggested by an autosomal recessive pattern in some families. The condition can readily be diagnosed sonographically by the characteristic 'double-bubble' appearance of the dilated stomach and proximal duodenum and the commonly associated polyhydramnios (Figure 1.24).

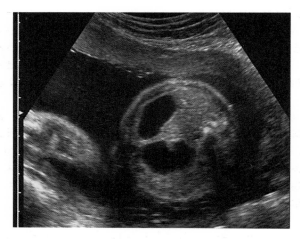

Figure 1.24 'Double-bubble' appearance of duodenal atresia in a 26 week fetus with trisomy 21.

However obstruction due to a central web may result in only a 'single bubble' representing the fluid-filled stomach. The ultrasonographic features of duodenal atresia usually develop after 24 weeks' gestation.

Postnatally, trisomy 21 is found in 20–30% of cases of duodenal atresia (Fonkalsrud *et al* 1969, Touloukian 1978). In prenatal series the mean frequency of chromosomal defects was 57% (Table 1.12)

Table 1.12 Reports on antenatally diagnosed duodenal atresia providing data on the gestation at diagnosis (GA), prevalence of chromosomal defects in the total group and in the subgroups with isolated duodenal atresia and those with additional abnormalities. 21 = trisomy 21

Author	N	GA	Chromosomal defects				
			Total	Isolated	Multiple	21	Other
Rizzo *et al* 90	10	?	60%	1/4	5/6	5	1
Nicolaides *et al* 92d	23	20-36	43%	1/6	9/17	10	-
Wilson *et al* 92	5	?	100%	3/3	2/2	3	1
Hsieh *et al* 92	3	?	67%	?	?	2	-
Gagnon *et al* 92	3	?	67%	-	2/3	1	-
Total	**44**	**20-36**	**57%**	**38%**	**64%**	**21**	**2**

Bowel obstruction

Jejunal and ileal obstructions are imaged as multiple, fluid-filled loops of bowel in the abdomen (Figure 1.25) and, in contrast to duodenal atresia, associated abnormalities are uncommon. In a combined series of 589 infants with jejunoileal atresia, there were five cases of Down syndrome (De Lorimier *et al* 1969).

Anorectal malformations are often associated with other abnormalities, usually of the genitourinary system. Large bowel obstruction can be diagnosed by the presence of fluid-filled loops of bowel in the lower abdomen without polyhydramnios. Anal atresia may not present any antenatally detectable sonographic features.

In a series of 24 fetuses with dilated bowel (including 14 cases of small and six cases of large bowel obstruction, and four cases of megacystis-microcolon-intestinal hypoperistalsis syndrome or myotonia dystrophica), the karyotype was normal in all but one case, in which the fetus had multiple other abnormalities (Nicolaides *et al* 1992d).

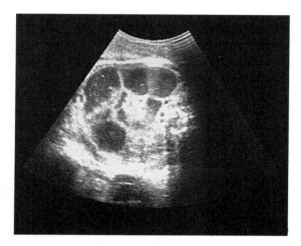

Figure 1.25 Dilated loop of bowel in a chromosomally normal 24 week fetus with small bowel obstruction.

Echogenic bowel

Hyperechogenic bowel (Figure 1.26) is found in 1 in 200 mid-trimester fetuses (Dicke & Crane 1992, Bromley *et al* 1994).

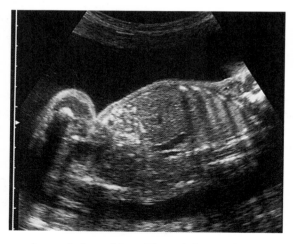

Figure 1.26 Hyperechogenic bowel in a 20 week fetus with trisomy 21.

This feature may be the consequence of intra-amniotic haemorrhage, severe uteroplacental insufficiency, cystic fibrosis and chromosomal defects. In four series reporting on hyperechogenic bowel in a total of 196 fetuses, 20% had chromosomal defects, mainly trisomy 21 (Table 1.13). Bromley *et al* (1994) estimated that 12.5% of fetuses with trisomy 21 have hyperechogenic bowel, that in 41% of these the echogenic bowel may be the only ultrasound finding and that the risk of Down syndrome in fetuses with isolated hyperechogenic bowel is 1.4%.

Table 1.13 Reports on the antenatal observation of hyperechogenic bowel providing data on the prevalence of chromosomal defects in the total group and in the subgroups where it was an isolated finding and those with additional abnormalities. GA = gestation in weeks, 21 = trisomy 21.

Author	N	GA	Chromosomal defects				
			Total	Isolated	Multiple	21	Other
Dicke & Crane 92	30	>14	3%	0/21	1/9	-	1
Scioscia *et al* 92	22	15-26	27%	2/17	4/5	5	1
Nyberg *et al* 93	95	>13	25%	7/60	17/35	11	13
Bromley *et al* 94	49	14-24	16%	0/31	6/18	6	2
Total	**196**	**13-26**	**20%**	**7%**	**42%**	**22**	**17**

In the Harris Birthright Research Centre for Fetal Medicine we observed hyperechogenic bowel in 280 fetuses and this was most commonly associated with placental insufficiency and intrauterine growth retardation; chromosomal defects were found only in those fetuses with additional, often multiple, abnormalities (Table 1.14).

Table 1.14 Prevalence of chromosomal defects in fetuses where hyperechogenic bowel was associated with (a) growth retardation, (b) minor abnormalities such as choroid plexus cyst, (c) major abnormalities. 21 = trisomy 21, 18 = trisomy 18, 13 = trisomy 13.

Group	N	Chromosomal defects					
		Total	21	18	13	Triploidy	Other
a. Growth retardation	91	0%	-	-	-	-	-
b. Minor abnormalities	122	2%	1	1	-	1	-
c. Major abnormalities	67	36%	6	6	6	2	4

Abdominal cysts

These include ovarian (Figure 1.27), mesenteric, adrenal and hepatic cysts. In a series of 27 fetuses with abdominal cysts the karyotype was normal in 26 cases; in one fetus with multiple adrenal cysts and hepatosplenomegaly due to the Beckwith-Wiedemann syndrome the karyotype was 46,XX/46,XX, dup(11p) (Nicolaides *et al* 1992d).

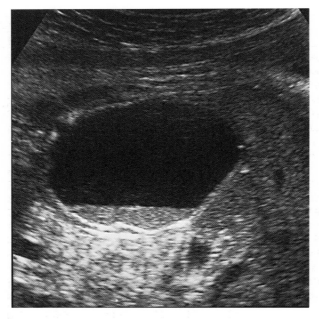

Figure 1.27 Haemorrhagic ovarian cyst in a 30 week chromosomally normal fetus.

Anterior abdominal wall abnormalities

Exomphalos

Exomphalos, with a birth incidence of about 1 per 3,000, is a correctable abnormality and when the condition is isolated postnatal survival is about 90%. It is associated with chromosomal defects and X-linked, autosomal dominant or autosomal recessive disorders. Prenatal diagnosis is based on the demonstration of the midline anterior abdominal wall defect, the herniated sac with its visceral contents and the umbilical cord insertion at the apex of the sac.

In liveborn infants with exomphalos, the prevalence of chromosomal defects, mainly trisomies 18 and 13 is approximately 10%
(see Chapter 2), whereas in antenatal series the reported
prevalence is about 36% (Table 1.15, Figure 1.28).

Table 1.15 Reports on the antenatal diagnosis of exomphalos providing data
on the prevalence of chromosomal defects in the total group and in those with
isolated exomphalos or additional abnormalities. 18 = trisomy 18, 13 = trisomy
13, Oth = other.

Author	N	GA	Chromosomal defects					
			Total	Isolated	Multiple	18	13	Oth
Nakayama *et al* 84	10	11-37	10%	1/4	0/6	1	-	-
Nicolaides *et al* 86	12	19-25	66%	1/3	7/9	7	-	1
Gilbert *et al* 87	35	16-36	54%	1/10	18/25	17	-	2
Sermer *et al* 87	10	15-40	40%	0/2	4/8	2	1	1
Edyoux *et al* 89	46	15-36	26%	7/27	5/19	6	2	4
Hughes *et al* 89	30	12-40	43%	3/8	10/22	4	5	4
Nyberg *et al* 89	26	12-30	38%	4/17	6/9	4	4	2
Benacerraf *et al* 90a	22	14-28	18%	0/7	4/15	1	2	1
Holzgreve *et al* 90	10	12-41	50%	?	?	3	1	1
Rizzo *et al* 90	12	15-38	58%	2/6	5/6	5	2	-
Getachew *et al* 91	22	15-34	23%	0/3	5/19	3	1	1
Rezai *et al* 91	24	12-40	29%	?	?	5	1	1
Van de Geijn *et al* 91	22	12-38	45%	0/4	10/18	6	1	3
Fogel *et al* 91	31	16-40	15%	0/14	5/17	3	1	1
Van Zalen-Sprock 91	18	11-38	39%	?	?	3	-	4
Nicolaides *et al* 92d	116	16-39	36%	0/30	41/86	32	7	3
Wilson *et al* 92	13	13-39	23%	0/7	2/6	3	-	-
Morrow *et al* 93	16	14-24	31%	3/?	2/?	3	-	2
Total	**475**	**11-41**	**35%**	**13%**	**46%**	**108**	**28**	**31**

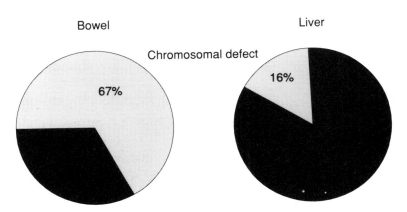

Figure 1.28 The frequency of chromosomal defects in fetuses with exomphalos
is 67% if the sac contains only bowel and 16% if the liver is also present.

The karyotype is more likely to be abnormal if the exomphalos is associated with additional abnormalities (46% compared to 13% for apparently isolated exomphalos). Furthermore, the frequency of chromosomal abnormalities is higher, when the exomphalos sac contains only bowel, than in cases where the liver is included (Figure 1.28; Hughes *et al* 1989, Nyberg *et al* 1989, Benacerraf *et al* 1990a, Getachew *et al* 1991, Nicolaides *et al* 1992d). The relationship between exomphalos and chromosomal defects is dealt with more extensively in Chapter 2.

Gastroschisis

In gastroschisis, with a birth incidence of 1 per 10,000, evisceration of the intestine occurs through a small abdominal wall defect located just lateral and usually to the right of an intact umbilical cord. Prenatal diagnosis is based on the demonstration of the normally situated umbilicus and the herniated loops of intestine, which are free-floating. The vast majority of cases are thought to be sporadic, although there are examples of familial gastroschisis suggesting the possibility of an autosomal dominant mode of inheritance, with variable expressivity. Associated chromosomal defects are rare, and although other abnormalities are found in 10–30% of the cases, these are mainly gut atresias, probably due to gut strangulation and infarction *in utero*. In four reports on a total of 63 fetuses with gastroschisis, there were no chromosomal defects (Van de Geijn *et al* 1991, Nicolaides *et al* 1992d, Wilson *et al* 1992, Morrow *et al* 1993).

Urinary tract abnormalities

Fetal urinary tract anomalies occur in approximately 2–3 per 1,000 pregnancies. Postnatal and postmortem studies have established that urinary tract defects are commonly found in many chromosomal defects (Jones *et al* 1988).

Prenatal series did not usually present data on the different types of renal defects and the overall prevalence of associated chromosomal abnormalities varied from 2% to 33%; the mean prevalence for isolated abnormalities was 3% and the prevalence for those with additional abnormalities was 24% (Table 1.16).

Table 1.16 Reports on the antenatally diagnosed renal abnormalities providing data on the prevalence of trisomies 21, 18 and 13 and other chromosomal defects in the total group and in the subgroups with isolated renal abnormalities and the group with additional abnormalities. Studies are classified under C according to the types of abnormalities into mixed (1), multicystic kidneys (2), obstruction (3), mild hydronephrosis (4). 21 = trisomy 21, 18 = trisomy 18, 13 = trisomy 13, Oth = other

Author	C	N	Chromosomal defects						
			Total	Isolated	Multiple	21	18	13	Oth
Nicolaides *et al* 86	1	45	24%	?	?	-	6	2	3
Rizzo *et al* 87	2	6	33%	0/3	2/3	-	-	1	1
Boue *et al* 88	1	221	11%	10/165	14/56	5	6	3	10
Hegge *et al* 88	1	3	33%	?	?	-	-	-	1
Reuss *et al* 88	3	43	12%	2/27	3/16	1	2	2	-
Eydoux *et al* 89	1	111	11%	1/55	11/56	2	4	3	3
Benacerraf *et al* 90b	4	210	3%	?	?	7	-	-	-
Holzgreve *et al* 90	1	16	25%	?	?	-	1	2	1
Rizzo *et al* 90	1	44	2%	1/44	0/0	-	-	-	1
Shah *et al* 90a	1	9	33%	?	?	1	-	1	1
Stoll *et al* 90	1	79	2%	?	?	4	6	4	7
Brumfield *et al* 91b	3	30	23%	5/25	2/5	-	2	2	3
Van Zalen-Sprock 91	4	21	5%	1/21	0/0	1	-	-	-
Nicolaides *et al* 92e	1	842	11%	9/452	87/360	23	25	20	28
Corteville *et al* 92	4	127	6%	0/116	7/11	4	-	-	3
Wilson *et al* 92	1	18	-	0/10	0/8	-	-	-	-
Total		**1825**	**11%**	**3%**	**24%**	**48**	**52**	**40**	**62**

In the largest series, renal abnormalities (Figure 1.29) were classified as (i) mild hydronephrosis, where only the renal pelvises are dilated and both the bladder and amniotic fluid volume are normal; (ii) moderate to severe hydronephrosis, with varying degrees of pelvic-calyceal dilatation; (iii) multicystic dysplasia, with multiple non-communicating cysts of variable size and irregular hyperechogenic stroma and (iv) renal agenesis (Nicolaides *et al* 1992b).

The renal abnormalities were either unilateral or bilateral. In the fetuses with bilateral moderate/severe hydronephrosis or multicystic kidneys, the obstruction was considered to be either low (if the bladder was dilated), or high (if the bladder was normal or empty) and there was either oligohydramnios or the amniotic fluid volume was normal/reduced.

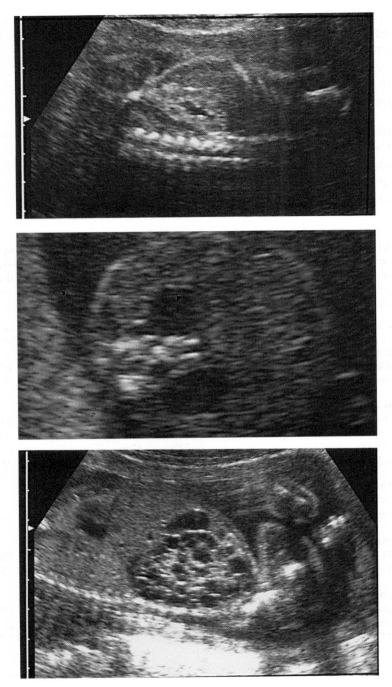

Figure 1.29 Renal abnormalities. Mild (top) and moderate (middle) hydronephrosis, and multicystic dysplasia (bottom).

The risk for chromosomal defects was similar for fetuses with unilateral or bilateral involvement, different types of renal abnormalities, urethral or ureteric obstruction, and oligohydramnios or normal/reduced amniotic fluid volume (Table 1.17). However, the prevalence of chromosomal defects in females was almost double (18%) that in males (10%).

The overall frequency of chromosomal defects was 12% and the most common were trisomies 21, 18 and 13. The pattern of chromosomal defects, and consequently that of associated malformations, was related to the different types of renal abnormalities (Table 1.18).

Table 1.17 Prevalence of chromosomal defects in fetuses with renal abnormalities in relation to the site and type of abnormality and fetal sex. For those with bilateral moderate/severe hydronephrosis or multicystic kidneys the frequency of chromosomal defects was examined in relation to the level of obstruction (high or ureteric and low or urethral) and amniotic fluid volume (modified from Nicolaides *et al* 1992b).

	N	Total	Isolated	Multiple
Renal abnormality - site				
Uniliteral	172	11%	2%	45%
Bilateral	510	13%	4%	31%
Renal abnormality - type				
Mild hydronephrosis	276	13%	3%	31%
Moderate/severe hydronephrosis	206	11%	4%	35%
Multicystic dysplasia	173	12%	3%	37%
Renal agenesis	27	15%	5%	38%
Fetal sex				
Male	492	10%	-	-
Female	190	18%	-	-
Obstruction				
High	67	9%	0%	29%
Low	156	14%	7%	33%
Amniotic fluid				
Oligohydramnios	120	12%	5%	36%
Normal/reduced	103	14%	5%	29%

Thus, in mild hydronephrosis, the commonest chromosomal defect was trisomy 21, whereas in moderate/severe hydronephrosis, multicystic kidneys, or renal agenesis the commonest defects were trisomies 18 and 13 each with their own syndromal abnormalities.

This study also demonstrated that, compared to the overall maternal age-related risk of the population examined, the risk for fetal chromosomal defects was three times higher when there was an apparently isolated renal abnormality and 30 times higher when there were additional malformations (Nicolaides *et al* 1992b). The possible significance of isolated mild hydronephrosis or pyelectasia is discussed further in Chapter 2.

Table 1.18 Frequency of chromosomal defects in relation to the type of renal abnormality. 21 = trisomy 21, 18 = trisomy 18, 13 = trisomy 13. Modified from Nicolaides *et al* 1992b.

Renal abnormality	N	Chromosomal defect			
		21	18	13	Other
Mild hydronephrosis	276	15	7	8	7
Moderate/severe hydronephrosis	206	3	4	5	11
Multicystic kidneys	173	1	8	4	8
Renal agenesis	27	-	1	1	2
Total	**682**	**19**	**20**	**18**	**28**

Skeletal abnormalities

There is a wide range of rare skeletal dyplasias, each with a specific recurrence risk, morphology and implication for neonatal survival and long-term prognosis (Jones *et al* 1988).

When an abnormality in the limbs and extremities is detected during a routine ultrasound examination, a systematic search is made for the detection of other defects that may lead to the diagnosis of a specific genetic syndrome. Similarly, chromosomal defects may be suspected from the presence of associated abnormalities.

Short femur

Benacerraf *et al* (1985) reported that, if the ratio of the actual femur length to the expected length, based on the biparietal diameter, was ≤ 0.91, the sensitivity and specificity for detecting fetuses with trisomy 21 at 15–21 weeks of gestation were 68% and 98%, respectively.

Subsequent studies have confirmed that trisomy 21 is associated with relative shortening of the femur but the sensitivity and specificity of this test were lower than those in the original report. In an additional five studies involving a total of 77 fetuses with trisomy 21, there was no significant difference in the mean biparietal diameter to femur length ratio and/or measured-to-expected femur ratio from that of normal controls (Winston & Horger 1988, La Follette *et al* 1989, Lynch *et al* 1989, Shah *et al* 1990b, Twining *et al* 1991a).

In a series of 155 fetuses with trisomy 21 diagnosed in the Harris Birthright Research Centre for Fetal Medicine, there was relative shortening of the femur, demonstrated by a head circumference to femur length ratio above the 97.5th centile, in 28% of the cases (Figure 1.30).

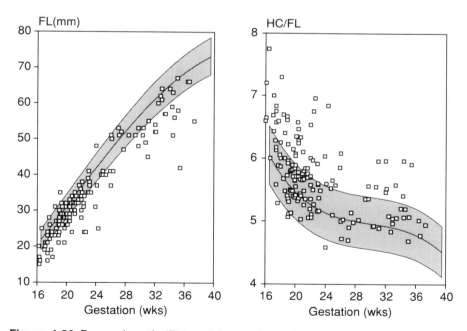

Figure 1.30 Femur length (FL) and head circumference to femur length ratio (HC/FL) in 155 fetuses with trisomy 21 diagnosed at the Harris Birthright Research Centre for Fetal Medicine plotted on the normal range for gestation (mean, 95th and 5th centiles).

In fetuses with trisomy 18, trisomy 13, triploidy and Turner syndrome, the prevalences of relative shortening of the femur were 25%, 9%, 60% and 59%, respectively (Figure 1.31).

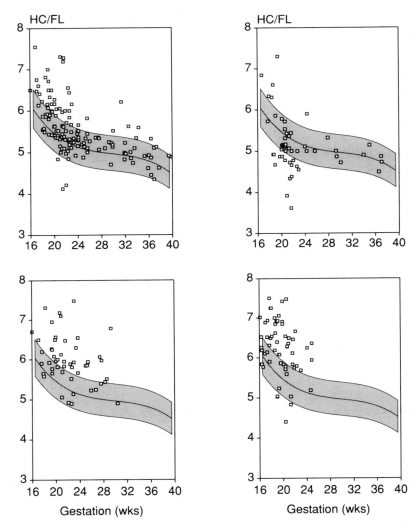

Figure 1.31 Head circumference to femur length ratio (HC/FL) in 137 fetuses with trisomy 18 (top, left), 54 with trisomy 13 (top, right), 50 with triploidy (bottom, left) and 65 with Turner syndrome (bottom, right) diagnosed at the Harris Birthright Research Centre for Fetal Medicine plotted on the normal range for gestation (mean, 95th and 5th centiles).

Short humerus

In a postmortem study of Down syndrome fetuses, FitzSimmons *et al* (1989) reported that shortening of the long bones of the upper extremity was more pronounced than that of the lower extremity. Four prenatal ultrasonographic studies at 15–22 weeks' of gestation have confirmed that in trisomy 21 there is relative shortening of the humerus, but they produced conflicting results as to the value of this feature in screening for trisomies (Table 1.19).

Table 1.19 Summary of reports on antenatally measured humerus length. Criteria (C) for diagnosis of short humerus were (1) a measurement below the 5th centile for gestation, or (2) a ratio of measured-to-expected of < 0.9 (2). GA = gestation in weeks, 21 = trisomy 21.

Author	C	GA	Controls	21	Sensitivity	Specificity
Rodis *et al* 91	1	15-22	1470	11	64%	95%
Benacerraf *et al* 91	2	14-20	400	24	50%	94%
Rotmensch *et al* 92	2	15-21	204	43	28%	91%
Biagiotti *et al* 94	2	15-19	500	27	56%	85%

Malformations of the extremities

Characteristic abnormalities in the extremities are commonly found in a wide range of chromosomal defects and the detection of abnormal hands or feet at the routine ultrasound examination should stimulate the search for other markers of chromosomal defects. Syndactyly is associated with triploidy, clinodactyly and sandal gap with trisomy 21, polydactyly with trisomy 13, and overlapping fingers, rocker bottom feet and talipes with trisomy 18 (Figures 1.32 and 1.33).

Talipes

Talipes equinovarus or calcaneovarus is a common abnormality found in 1–2 per 1,000 live births (Figure 1.33). In the majority of cases the aetiology is uncertain but in some families an autosomal recessive mode of inheritance has been described.

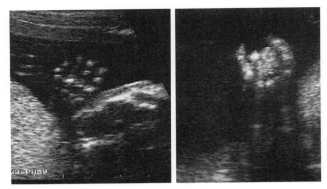

Figure 1.32 Clinodactyly of the fifth finger in a fetus with trisomy 21 (left) and overlapping fingers in a fetus with trisomy 18 (right).

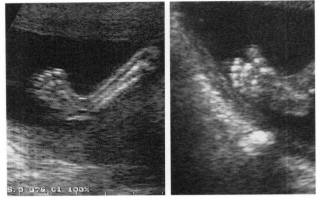

Figure 1.33 Talipes in a fetus with trisomy 18 (left) and 'sandal gap' in a fetus with trisomy 21 (right).

In 243 fetuses with talipes examined at the Harris Birthright Research Centre for Fetal Medicine, only 22% of the cases had isolated talipes. In the others, the talipes was associated with (i) chromosomal defects, (ii) neural tube or brain abnormalities, (iii) oligohydramnios due to renal abnormalities or preterm prelabour amniorrhexis, (iv) skeletal dysplasias such as osteogenesis imperfecta, or (v) arthrogryposis, where, in addition to the talipes, there was fixed flexion or extension deformity of all major joints.

In three series on a total of 127 cases of antenatally diagnosed talipes equinovarus, 33% had chromosomal defects, mainly trisomy 18 (Jeanty *et al* 1985, Benacerraf 1986b, Nicolaides *et al* 1992e). All the fetuses with chromosomal defects had multiple abnormalities.

Intrauterine growth retardation

Although low birth weight is a common feature of many chromosomal defects, the frequency of chromosomal defects in small for gestational age neonates is less than 1–2% (Chen *et al* 1972, Ounsted *et al* 1981, Khoury *et al* 1988). However, data derived from postnatal studies underestimate the association between chromosomal defects and growth retardation, since many pregnancies with chromosomally abnormal fetuses result in spontaneous abortion or intrauterine death. Furthermore, since the degree of growth retardation is generally more severe in the more lethal types of chromosomal defects, in antenatally diagnosed, early onset, severe growth retardation the types of chromosomal defects are different from those recognised at birth.

In two prenatal series reporting on a total of 621 growth retarded fetuses, the prevalence of chromosomal defects was 19% (Table 1.20).

Table 1.20 Fetal karyotype in 621 growth retarded fetuses at 17–40 weeks of gestation. 18 = trisomy 18, 13 = trisomy 13, Trip = triploidy, Oth = other.

Author	N	Chromosomal defects						
		Total	Isolated	Multiple	18	13	Trip	Oth
Eydoux *et al* 89	163	17%	10/106	17/57	15	6	1	5
Snijders *et al* 93	458	19%	4/243	85/215	32	5	35	13
Total	**621**	**19%**	**4%**	**38%**	**47**	**11**	**36**	**18**

Snijders *et al* (1993) examined findings in 458 fetuses with an abdominal circumference and subsequently birth weight below the 5th centile for gestation (Figure 1.34). The commonest chromosomal defects were triploidy and trisomy 18. The characteristic Swiss-cheese appearance of a molar placenta was found in only 17% of fetuses with triploidy; in the others the placenta looked normal and the main feature was severe asymmetrical growth retardation. The triploidies were most commonly encountered in the second trimester while the aneuploidies, deletions and translocations were found in the third trimester group of fetuses. These findings suggest that triploidy is associated with the most severe form of early-onset growth retardation and that most affected fetuses die before the third trimester of pregnancy.

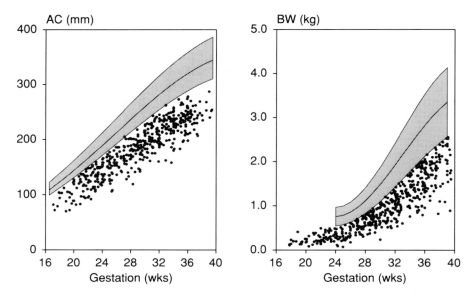

Figure 1.34 Abdominal circumference (AC) and birth weight (BW) of the 458 growth retarded fetuses plotted on the appropriate reference range (mean, 95th and 5th centiles) for gestation (Snijders *et al* 1993).

The highest frequency of chromosomal defects was found in those cases where, in addition to the growth retardation, there were fetal structural abnormalities, the amniotic fluid volume was normal or increased and those with normal waveforms from both uterine and umbilical arteries (Table 1.21).

These findings demonstrate that growth retardation due to chromosomal defects presents differently from growth retardation due to placental insufficiency. The latter is characterised by increased impedance to flow in the uterine and/or umbilical arteries, with consequent fetal hypoxemia, redistribution in the fetal circulation, impaired renal perfusion, and reduced urine production and amniotic fluid volume.

It is generally assumed that fetal causes of growth retardation, such as chromosomal defects, are associated with early-onset, symmetrical impairment in growth of all parts of the body. In contrast, placental insufficiency is associated with late-onset, asymmetrical impairment in growth, primarily affecting the abdomen and sparing the head and femur. However, the study of Snijders *et al* (1993) demonstrated that relative shortening of the femur is found in both the chromosomally normal and abnormal fetuses (Figure 1.35).

Table 1.21 Frequency of chromosomal defects in 458 growth retarded fetuses in relation to gestation at presentation, the presence of fetal abnormalities, amniotic fluid volume and Doppler findings (absence or presence of an early diastolic notch in the waveforms from the uterine arteries and presence or absence of end-diastolic frequencies (EDF) in the waveforms from the umbilical arteries).

Feature	N	Chromosomal defects
Gestation at presentation		
18–25 wks	132	38%
26–33 wks	208	10%
34–41 wks	118	15%
Additional fetal abnormalities		
Present	215	40%
Absent	143	3%
Amniotic fluid volume		
Increased	20	95%
Normal	147	32%
Reduced	159	10%
Absent	132	5%
Doppler findings		
No notch / EDF +ve	111	44%
No notch / EDF - ve	46	24%
Notch / EDF +ve	113	12%
Notch / EDF - ve	188	8%

Fetuses with triploidy have severe, early-onset, asymmetrical growth retardation (increased head to abdomen circumference ratio), whereas fetuses with chromosomal defects other than triploidy are symmetrically growth retarded before 30 weeks, but those diagnosed after this gestation are usually asymmetrically growth retarded (Figure 1.35).

Since in normal pregnancy the head to abdomen circumference ratio decreases with gestation, it could be postulated that chromosomal defects interfere with the developmental clock that controls the switch from preferential growth of the head to growth of the abdomen.

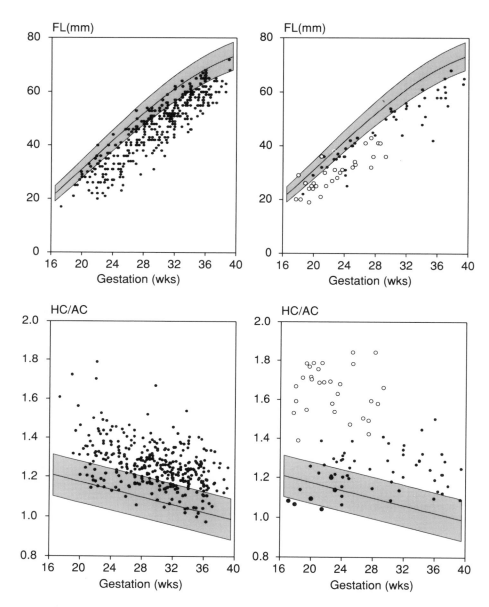

Figure 1.35 Femur length (FL) and head to abdomen circumference ratio (HC/AC) in chromosomally normal (left) and abnormal (right; ○ =triploidy with molar placenta, ●=triploidy with normal placenta, ■=trisomies) growth retarded fetuses plotted on the appropriate reference range (mean, 95th and 5th centiles) for gestation (Snijders *et al* 1993).

REFERENCES

Aase JM, Wilson AC, Smith DW. Small ears in Down's syndrome: a helpful diagnostic aid. J Pediatr 1973;82:845.

Abramowicz JS, Warsof SL, Doyle DL, Smith D, Levy DL. Congenital cystic hygroma of the neck diagnosed prenatally: outcome with normal and abnormal karyotype. Prenat Diagn 1989;9:321-7.

Achiron R, Barkai G, Katznelson MBM, Mashiach S. Fetal lateral ventricle choroid plexus cysts: the dilemma of amniocentesis. Obstet Gynecol 1991;78:815-18.

Allan LD, Sharland GK, Chita SK, Lockhart S, Maxwell DJ. Chromosomal anomalies in fetal congenital heart disease. Ultrasound Obstet Gynecol 1991;1:8-11.

Allan LD, Sharland GK, Milburn A, Lockhart SM, Groves AM, Anderson RH, Cook AC, Fagg NLK. Prospective diagnosis of 1,006 consecutive cases of congenital heart disease in the fetus. J Am Coll Cardiol 1994;23:1452-8.

Anhoury P, Andre M, Droulle P, Czorny A, Gilgenkrantz S, Schweitzer M, Leheup B. Dilatation des ventricules cerebraux decouverte in utero. A propos de 85 observations. J Gynecol Obstet Biol Reprod 1991;20:191-7.

Awwad JT, Azar GB, Karam KS, Nicolaides KH. Ear length: a potential sonographic marker for Down syndrome. Int J Gynecol Obstet 1994;44:233-8.

Azar G, Snijders RJM, Gosden CM, Nicolaides KH. Fetal nuchal cystic hygromata: associated malformations and chromosomal defects. Fetal Diagn Ther 1991;6:46-57.

Bahado-Singh RO, Wyse L, Dorr MA, Copel JA, O'Connor T, Hobbins J. Fetuses with Down syndrome have disproportionately shortened frontal lobe dimensions on ultrasonographic examination. Am J Obstet Gynecol 1992;167:1009-14.

Benacerraf BR, Barss VA, Laboda LA. A sonographic sign for the detection in the second trimester of the fetus with Down's syndrome. Am J Obstet Gynecol 1985;151:1078-9.

Benacerraf BR, Frigoletto FD, Green MF. Abnormal facial features and extremities in human trisomy syndromes: prenatal US appearance. Radiology 1986a;159:243-6.

Benacerraf BR. Antenatal sonographic diagnosis of congenital clubfoot: a possible indication for amniocentesis. J Clin Ultrasound 1986b;14:703-6.

Benacerraf BR, Adzick NS. Fetal diaphragmatic hernia: ultrasound diagnosis and clinical outcome in 19 cases. Am J Obstet Gynecol 1987a;156:573-6.

Benacerraf BR, Gelman R, Frigoletto FD. Sonographic identification of second trimester fetuses with Down's syndrome. N Engl J Med 1987b;317:1371-6.

Benacerraf BR, Laboda LA. Cyst of the fetal choroid plexus: a normal variant. Am J Obstet Gynecol 1989;160:319-21.

Benacerraf BR, Saltzman DH, Estroff JH, Frigoletto FD Jr. Abnormal karyotype of fetuses with omphalocele: prediction based on omphalocele contents. Obstet Gynecol 1990a;75:317-19.

Benacerraf BR, Mandell J, Estroff JA, Harlow BL, Frigoletto FD Jr. Fetal pyelectasis: a possible association with Down Syndrome. Obstet Gynecol 1990b;76:58-60.

Benacerraf BR, Neuberg D, Frigoletto FD Jr. Humeral shortening in second trimester fetuses with Down Syndrome. Obstet Gynecol 1991;77:223-7.

Benacerraf BR, Laboda LA, Frigoletto FD. Thickened nuchal fold in fetuses not at risk for aneuploidy. Radiology 1992;184:239-42.

Benacerraf BR, Mulliken JB. Fetal cleft lip and palate: sonographic diagnosis and postnatal outcome. Plast Reconstr Surg 1993;92:1045.

Bernard P, Chabaud JJ, Le Guern H, Le Bris MJ, Boog G. Hygroma kystique du cou. Diagnostic antenatal, facteurs pronostiques, conduite a tenir. A propos de 42 cas. J Gynecol Obstet Biol Reprod 1991;20:487-95.

Berry SM, Gosden CM, Snijders RJM, Nicolaides KH. Fetal holoprosencephaly: associated malformations and chromosomal defects. Fetal Diagn Ther 1990;5:92-9.

Biagiotti R, Periti E, Cariati E. Humerus and femur length in fetuses with Down syndrome. Pren Diagn 1994;14:429-34.

Birnholz JC, Farrell EE. Fetal ear length. Pediatrics 1988;81:555-8.

Blake DM, Copel JA, Kleinman CS. Hypoplastic left heart syndrome: prenatal diagnosis, clinical profile, and management. Am J Obstet Gynecol 1991;165:529-34.

Boue A, Muller F, Briard ML, Boue J. Interest of biology in the management of pregnancies where a fetal malformation has been detected by ultrasonography. Fetal Ther 1988;3:14-23.

Bromley B, Frigoletto Jr FD, Benacerraf BR. Mild fetal lateral cerebral ventriculomegaly: clinical course and outcome. Am J Obstet Gynecol 1991;164:863-7.

Bromley B, Doubilet P, Frigoletto Jr FD, Krauss C, Estroff JA, Benacerraf BR. Is fetal hyperechoic bowel on second-trimester sonogram an indication for amniocentesis? Obstet Gynecol 1994;83:647-51.

Bronshtein M, Blumenfeld I, Kohn J, Blulmenfeld Z. Detection of cleft lip by early second-trimester transvaginal sonography. Obstet Gynecol 1994;84:73-6.

Brown DL, Roberts DJ, Miller WA. Left ventricular echogenic focus in the fetal heart: pathologic correlation. J Ultrasound Med 1994;13:613-16.

Brumfield CG, Davis RO, Hauth JC, Cosper P, Colvin EV, Finley S. Management of prenatally detected nonlethal fetal anomalies: is a karyotype of benefit? Am J Perinat 1991a;8:255-8.

Brumfield CG, Davis RO, Joseph DB, Cosper P. Fetal obstructive uropathies: importance of chromosomal abnormalities and associated anomalies to perinatal outcome. J Reprod Med 1991b;36:662-6.

Byrne J, Blanc W, Warburton D, Wigger J. The significance of cystic hygroma in fetuses. Hum Pathol 1984;15:61-7.

Carr RF, Ochs RH, Ritter DA, Kenny JD, Fridey JL, Ming PL. Fetal cystic hygroma and Turner's syndrome. Am J Dis Child 1986;140:580-3.

Chan L, Hixson JL, Laifer SA, Marchese SG, Martin JG, Hill LM. A sonographic and karyotypic study of second trimester fetal choroid plexus cysts. Obstet Gynecol 1989;73:703-5.

Chen ATL, Chan YK, Falek A. The effects of chromosomal abnormalities on birth weight in man. Human Heredity 1972:209-24.

Chervenak FA, Isaacson G, Blakemore KJ, Breg RW, Hobbins JC, Berkowitz RL, Tortora M, Mayden K, Mahoney MJ. Fetal cystic hygroma: cause and natural history. N Engl J Med 1983;309:822-5.

Chervenak FA, Berkowitz RL, Tortora M, Hobbins JC. The management of fetal hydrocephalus. Am J Obstet Gynecol 1985a;151:933-42.

Chervenak FA, Isaacson G, Hobbins JC, Chitkara U, Tortora M, Berkowitz RL. Diagnosis and management of fetal holoprosencephaly. Obstet Gynecol 1985b;66:322-6.

Chinn DH, Miller EI, Worthy LM, Towers CV. Sonographically detected fetal choroid plexus cysts: frequency and association with aneuploidy. J Ultrasound Med 1991;10:255-8.

Chitkara U, Cogswell C, Norton K, Wilkins IA, Mehalek K, Berkowitz RL. Choroid plexus cysts in the fetus: a benign anatomic variant or pathologic entity? Report of 41 cases and review of the literature. Obstet Gynecol 1988;72:185-9.

Clark SL, De Vore GR, Sabey PL. Prenatal diagnosis of cysts of the fetal choroid plexus. Obstet Gynecol 1988;72:585-7.

Cochrane DD, Myles ST, Nimrod C, Still DK, Sugarman RG, Wittmann BK. Intrauterine hydrocephalus and ventriculomegaly: associated abnormalities and fetal outcome. Can J Neurol Sci 1985;12:51-9.

Comstock C, Culp D, Gonzalez J, Boal DB. Agenesis of the corpus callosum in the fetus: its evolution and significance. J Ultrasound Med 1985;4:613-16.

Corteville JE, Dicke JM, Crane JP. Fetal pyelectasis and Down syndrome: is genetic amniocentesis warranted? Obstet Gynecol 1992;79:770-2.

Crane J, Gray D. Sonographically measured nuchal skinfold thickness as a screening tool for Down syndrome: results of a prospective clinical trial. Obstet Gynecol 1991;77:533-6.

DeLorimier AA, Fonkalsrud EW, Hays DM. Congenital atresia and stenosis of the jejunum and ileum. Surgery 1969;65:819-27.

DeRoo TR, Harris RD, Sargent SK, Denholm TA, Crow HC. Fetal choroid plexus cysts: prevalence, clinical significance and sonographic appearence. Am J Roentgenol 1988;151:1179-81.

DeVore GR, Alfi O. The association between an abnormal nuchal skin fold, trisomy 21, and ultrasound abnormalities identified during the second trimester of pregnancy. Ultrasound Obstet Gynecol 1993;3:387-94.

Dicke JM, Crane JP. Sonographically detected hyperechoic fetal bowel: significance and implications for pregnancy management. Obstet Gynecol 1992;80:778-82.

Donnenfeld AE, Carlson DE, Palomaki GE, Librizzi RJ, Weiner S, Platt L. Prospective multicenter study of second-trimester nuchal skinfold thickness in unaffected and Down syndrome pregnancies. Obstet Gynecol 1994;84:844-7.

Drugan A, Krause B, Canady A, Zador IE, Sacks AJ, Evans MI. The natural history of prenatally diagnosed cerebral ventriculomegaly. J Am Med Assoc 1989;261:1785-8.

Estroff JA, Scott MR, Benacerraf BR. Dandy-Walker variant: prenatal sonographic features and clinical outcome. Radiology 1992;185:755-8.

Eydoux P, Choiset A, Le Porrier N, Thepot F, Szpiro-tapia S, Alliet J, Ramond S, Viel JF, Gautier E, Morichon N, Girard-Orgeolet S. Chromosomal prenatal diagnosis: study of 936 cases of intrauterine abnormalities after ultrasound assessment. Prenat Diagn 1989;9:255-68.

Filly RA, Chin DH, Callen PW. Alobar holoprosencephaly: ultrasonographic prenatal diagnosis. Radiology 1984;151:455-9.

Fogel M, Copel JA, Cullen MT, Hobbins JC, Kleinman CS. Congenital heart disease and fetal thoracoabdominal anomalies: association in utero and the importance of cytogenetic analysis. Am J Perinatol 1991;8:411-16.

Fonkalsrud EW, DeLorimier AA, Hays DM. Congenital atresia and stenosis of the duodenum. A review compiled from the members of the surgical section of the American Academy of Pediatrics. Pediatrics 1969;43:79-83.

FitzSimmons J, Droste S, Shepard TH, Pascoe-Manson J, Chinn A, Mack LA. Long bone growth in fetuses with Down syndrome. Am J Obstet Gynecol 1989;161:1174-7.

Gabrielli S, Reece AR, Pilu G, Perolo A, Rizzo N, Bovicelli L, Hobbins JC. The significance of prenatally diagnosed choroid plexus cysts. Am J Obstet Gynecol 1989;160:1207-10.

Gagnon S, Fraser W, Fouquette B, Bastide A, Bureau M, Fontaine JY, Hout C. Nature and frequency of chromosomal abnormalities in pregnancies with abnormal ultrasound findings: an analysis of 117 cases with review of the literature. Prenat Diagn 1992;12:9-18.

German JC, Mahour GH, Wooley MM. Esophageal atresia and associated anomalies. J Pediatr Surg 1976;11:299-306.

Getachew MM, Goldstein RB, Edge V, Golberg JD, Filly RA. Correlation between omphalocele contents and karyotypic abnormalities: sonographic study in 37 cases. Am J Roentgenol 1991;158:133-6.

Gilbert WM, Nicolaides KH. Fetal omphalocele: associated malformations and chromosomal defects. Obstet Gynecol 1987;70:633-5.

Hegge FN, Prescott GH, Watson PT. Sonography at the time of genetic amniocentesis to screen for fetal malformations. Obstet Gynecol 1988;71:522-5.

Hertzberg BS, Kay HH, Bowie JD. Fetal choroid plexus lesions: relationship of antenatal sonographic appearence to clinical outcome. J Ultrasound Med 1989;8:77-82.

Holzgreve W, Miny P, Gerlach B, Westendorp A, Ahlert D, Horst J. Benefits of placental biopsies for rapid karyotyping in the second and third trimesters (late chorionic villus sampling) in high-risk pregnancies. Am J Obstet Gynecol 1990;162:1188-92.

Holzgreve W, Feiel R, Louwen F, Miny P. Prenatal diagnosis and management of fetal hydrocephaly and lissencephaly. Child Nerv Syst 1993;9:408-12.

How HY, Villafane J, Parihus RR, Spinnato JA. Small hyperechoic foci of the fetal cardiac ventricle: a benign sonographic finding? Ultrasound Obstet Gynecol 1994;4:205-7.

Howard RJ, Tuck SM, Long J, Thomas VA. The significance of choroid plexus cysts in fetuses at 18-20 weeks. An indication for amniocentesis? Prenat Diagn 1992;12:685-8.

Hsieh FJ, Lee CN, Wu CC, Ko TM, Kao ML, Wong AH, Chen ML, Chen HY. Antenatal ultrasonic findings of craniofacial malformations. J Formosan Med Assoc 1991;90:551-4.

Hsieh FJ, Ko TM, Tseng LH, Chang LS, Pan MF, Chuang SM, Lee TY, Chen HY. Prenatal cytogenetic diagnosis in amniocentesis. J Formosan Med Assoc 1992;91:276-82.

Hudgins RJ, Edwards MSB, Goldstein R, Callen PW, Harrison MR, Filly RA, Golbus MS. Natural history of fetal ventriculomegaly. Pediatrics 1988;82:692-7.

Hughes M, Nyberg DH, Mack LH, Pretorius DH. Fetal omphalocele: prenatal US detection of concurrent anomalies and other predictors of outcome. Radiology 1989;173:371-6.

Jauniaux E, Maldergem LV, Munter CD, Moscoso G, Gillerot Y. Nonimmune hydrops fetalis associated with genetic abnormalities. Obstet Gynecol 1990;75:568-72.

Jeanty P, Romero R, d'Alton M, Venus I, Hobbins JC. In utero sonographic detection of hand and foot deformities. J Ultrasound Med 1985;4:595-601.

Jones KL. Smith's recognizable patterns of human malformation. 4th ed. London, WB Saunders 1988.

Khoury MJ, Erickson JD, Cordero JF, McCarthy BJ. Congenital malformations and intrauterine growth retardation: a population study. Pediatrics 1988;82:83-90.

Kirk JS, Comstock CH, Fassnacht MA, Yang SS, Lee W. Routine measurement of nuchal thickness in the second trimester. J Matern Fetal Med 1992;1:82-6.

LaFollette L, Filly RA, Anderson R, Golbus M. Fetal femur length to detect trisomy 21. A reappraisal. J Ultrasound Med 1989;8:657-60.

Lettieri L, Rodis JF, Vintzileos AM, Feeney L, Ciarleglio L, Craffey A. Ear length in second-trimester aneuploid fetuses. Obstet Gynecol 1993;81:57-60.

Lockwood CJ, Ghidini A, Aggarwal R, Hobbins J. Antenatal diagnosis of partial agenesis of the corpus callosum: a benign cause of ventriculomegaly. Am J Obstet Gynecol 1988;159:184-6.

Louhimo I, Lindahl H. Esophageal atresia: primary results of 500 consecutively treated patients. J Pediatr Surg 1983;18:217-29.

Lynch L, Berkowitz GS, Chitkara U, Wilkins IA, Mehalek KE, Berkowitz RL. Ultrasound detection of Down syndrome: is it really possible? Obstet Gynecol 1989;73:267-70.

MacLeod AM, McHugo MB. Prenatal diagnosis of nuchal cystic hygroma. Br J Radiol 1991;64:802-7.

Marchese C, Savin E, Dragone E, Carozzi F, De Marchi M, Campogrande M, Dolfin GC, Pagliano G, Viora E, Carbonara A. Cystic hygroma: prenatal diagnosis and genetic counselling. Prenat Diagn 1985;5:221-7.

Matsunaga E, Shiota K. Holoprosencephaly in human embryos: epidemiologic studies of 150 cases. Teratology 1977;16:261-72.

Miyabara S, Sugihara H, Maehara N, Shouno H, Tasaki H, Yoshida K, Saito N, Kayama F, Ibara S, Suzumori K. Significance of cardiovascular malformations in cystic hygroma: a new interpretation of the pathogenesis. Am J Med Genet 1989;34:489-501.

Morrow RJ, Whittle MJ, McNay MB, Raine PAM, Gibson AAM, Crossley J. Prenatal diagnosis and management of anterior abdominal wall defects in the west of Scotland. Prenat Diagn 1993;13:111-15.

Nadel AS, Bromley BS, Frigoletto FD Jr, Estroff JA, Benacerraf BR. Isolated choroid plexus cysts in the second-trimester fetus: is amniocentesis really indicated? Radiology 1992;185:545-8.

Nakayama DK, Harrison MK, Gross BH, Callen PW, Filly RH, Golbus MS, Stephens JU, de-Lorimier HH. Management of the fetus with an abdominal wall defect. J Pediatr Surg 1984;19:408-13.

Nava S, Godmilow L, Reeser S, Ludominky A, Donnenfeld AE. Significance of sonographically detected second trimester choroid plexus cysts: a series of 211 cases and a review of the literature. Ultrasound Obstet Gynecol 1994;4:448-51.

Newman DE, Cooperberg Pl. Genetics of sonographically detected intrauterine fetal cystic hygromas. J Can Assoc Radiol 1984;35:77-9.

Nicolaides KH, Rodeck CH, Lange I, Watson J, Gosden CM, Miller D, Mibashan RS, Moniz C, Morgan-Capner P, Campbell S. Fetoscopy in the assessment of unexplained fetal hydrops. Br J Obstet Gynaecol 1985;92:671-9.

Nicolaides KH, Rodeck CH, Gosden CM. Rapid karyotyping in non-lethal fetal malformations. Lancet 1986 i:283-7.

Nicolaides KH, Berry S, Snijders RJM, Thorpe-Beeston JG, Gosden CM. Fetal lateral cerebral ventriculomegaly: associated malformations and chromosomal defects. Fetal Diagn Ther 1990;5:5-14.

Nicolaides KH, Azar G, Snijders RJM, Gosden CM. Fetal nuchal edema: associated malformations and chromosomal defects. Fetal Diagn Ther 1992a;7:123-31.

Nicolaides KH, Cheng H, Abbas A, Snijders RJM, Gosden CM. Fetal renal defects: associated malformations and chromosomal defects. Fetal Diagn Ther 1992b;7:1-11.

Nicolaides KH, Salvesen D, Snijders RJM, Gosden CM. Strawberry shaped skull: associated malformations and chromosomal defects. Fetal Diagn Ther 1992c;7:132-7.

Nicolaides KH, Snijders RJM, Cheng H, Gosden CM. Fetal gastrointestinal and abdominal wall defects: associated malformations and chromosomal defects. Fetal Diagn Ther 1992d;7:102-15.

Nicolaides KH, Snijders RJM, Gosden CM, Berry C, Campbell S. Ultrasonographically detectable markers of fetal chromosomal abnormalities. Lancet 1992e;340:704-7.

Nicolaides KH, Salvesen DR, Snijders RJM, Gosden CM. Fetal facial defects: associated malformations and chromosomal abnormalities. Fetal Diagn Ther 1993;8:1-9.

Nora JJ, Nora AH. The evolution of specific genetic and environmental counseling in congenital heart disease. Circulation 1978;57:205-13.

Nyberg DA, Mack LA, Hirsch J, Pagon R, Shepard TH. Fetal hydrocephalus: sonographic detection and clinical significance of associated anomalies. Radiology 1987a;163:187-91.

Nyberg DA, Mack LA, Bronstein A, Hirsch J, Pagon RA. Holoprosencephaly: prenatal sonographic diagnosis. Am J Roentgenol 1987b;149:1051-8.

Nyberg DA, FitzSimmons J, Mack LH, Hughes M, Pretorius DH, Hickok D, Shepard IH. Chromosomal abnormalities in fetuses with omphalocele: significance of omphalocele contents. J Ultrasound Med 1989;8:299-308.

Nyberg DA, Resta RG, Luthy DA. Prenatal sonographic findings of Down syndrome: review of 94 cases. Obstet Gynecol 1990;76:370-7.

Nyberg DA, Mahony BS, Hegge FN, Hickok DE, Luthy DA, Kapur R. Enlarged cisterna magna and the Dandy-Walker malformation: factors associated with chromosome abnormalities. Obstet Gynecol 1991;77:436-42.

Nyberg DA, Dubinsky TD, Resta RG, Mahony BS, Hickok DE, Luthy DA. Echogenic fetal bowel during the second trimester: clinical importance. Radiology 1993;188:527-31.

Oettinger M, Odeh M, Korenblum R, Markovits J. Antenatal diagnosis of choroid plexus cyst: suggested management. Obstet Gynecol Surv 1993;48: 635-9.

Ostlere SJ, Irving HC, Lilford RJ. A prospective study of the incidence and significance of fetal choroid plexus cysts. Prenat Diagn 1990;9:205-11.

Ounsted M, Moar V, Scott A. Perinatal morbidity and mortality in small-for-dates babies: the relative importance of some maternal factors. Early Human Development 1981;5:367-75.

Paladini D, Calabro R, Palmieri S, D'Andrea T. Prenatal diagnosis of congenital heart disease and fetal karyotyping. Obstet Gynecol 1993;81:679-82.

Palmer CG, Miles JH, Howard-Peebles PN, Magenis RE, Patil S, Friedman JM. Fetal karyotype following ascertainment of fetal anomalies by ultrasound. Prenat Diagn 1987;7:551-5.

Pashayan HM. What else to look for in a child born with a cleft of the lip or palate. Cleft Palate J 1983;20:54-82.

Pearce MJ, Griffin D, Campbell S. The differential prenatal diagnosis of cystic hygromata and encephalocele by ultrasound examination. J Clin Ultrasound 1985;13:317-20.

Perpignano MC, Cohen HL, Klein VR, Mandel FS, Streltzoff J, Chervenak FA, Goldman MA. Fetal choroid plexus cysts: beware the smaller cyst. Radiology 1992;182:715-17.

Perrella R, Duerinckx AJ, Grant EG, Tessler F, Tabsh K, Crandall BF. Second trimester sonographic diagnosis of Down syndrome: role of femur length shortening and nuchal-fold thickening. Am J Roentgenol 1988;151:981-5.

Perry TB, Benzie RJ, Cassar N. Fetal cephalometry by ultrasound as a screening procedure for the prenatal detection of Down syndrome. Br J Obstet Gynaecol 1984;91:138-43.

Pilu G, Rizzo N, Orsini LF, Bovicelli L. Antenatal recognition of cerebral anomalies. Ultrasound Med Biol 1986;12:319-26.

Platt LD, Carlson DE, Medearis AL, Walla CA. Fetal choroid plexus cysts in the second trimester of pregnancy: a cause of concern. Am J Obstet Gynecol 1991;164:1652-6.

Porto M, Murata Y, Warneke LA, Keegan KA Jr. Fetal choroid plexus cysts: an independent risk factor for chromosomal anomalies. J Clin Ultrasound 1993;21:103-8.

Rebaud A, Chardon C, Rebaud MF, Berland M. Depistage antenatal des kystes des plexus choroides - Evolution et interpretation de 30 observations. J Gynecol Obstet Biol Reprod 1992;21:665-70.

Redford DHA, Mcnay MB, Ferguson-Smith ME, Jamieson ME. Aneuploidy and cystic hygroma detectable by ultrasound. Prenat Diagn 1984;4:377-82.

Reuss A, Wladimiroff JW, Stewart PA, Scholtmeijer RJ. Non-invasive mangement of fetal obstructive uropathy. Lancet 1988;ii:949-51.

Rezai K, Holzgreve W, Schloo R, Tercanli S, Horst J, Miny P. Pranatale Chromosomenbefunde bei sonographisch auffalligen Feten. Geburtsh Frauenh 1991;51:211-16.

Ricketts NEM, Lowe EM, Patel NB. Prenatal diagnosis of choroid plexus cysts. Lancet 1987;1:213-14.

Rizzo N, Gabrielli S, Pilu G, Perolo A, Cacciari A, Domini R, Bovicelli L. Prenatal diagnosis and obstetrical management of multicystic dysplastic kidney disease. Prenat Diagn 1987;7:109-18.

Rizzo N, Pitalis MC, Pilu G, Orsini LF, Perolo A, Bovicelli L. Prenatal karyotyping in malformed fetuses. Prenat Diagn 1990;10:17-23.

Rodis JF, Vintzileos AM, Fleming AD, Ciarleglio L, Nardi DA, Feeney L, Scorza WE, Campbell WA, Ingardia C. Comparison of humerus length with femur length in fetuses with Down Syndrome. Am J Obstet Gynecol 1991;165:1051-6.

Rotmensch S, Luo JS, Liberati M, Belanger K, Mahoney MJ, Hobbins JC. Fetal humeral length to detect Down Syndrome. Am J Obstet Gynecol 1992;166:1330-4.

Saltzman DH, Benacerraf BR, Frigoletto FD. Diagnosis and management of fetal facial clefts. Am J Obstet Gynecol 1986;155:377-9.

Scioscia AL, Pretorius DH, Budorick NE, Cahill TC, Axelrod FT, Leopold GR. Second trimester echogenic bowel and chromosomal abnormalities. Am J Obstet Gynecol 1992;167:889-94.

Sermer M, Benzie RJ, Pitson L, Carr M, Skidmore M. Prenatal diagnosis and management of congenital defects of the anterior abdominal wall. Am J Obstet Gynecol 1987;156:308-12.

Shah DM, Roussis P, Ulm J, Jeanty P, Boehm FH. Cordocentesis for rapid karyotyping. Am J Obstet Gynecol 1990a;162:1548-53.

Shah YG, Eckl CJ, Stinson SK, Woods JR. Biparietal diameter/femur length ratio, cephalic index, and femur length measurements: not reliable screening techniques for Down syndrome. Obstet Gynecol 1990b;75:186-8.

Sharland GK, Lockhart SM, Heward AJ, Allan LD. Prognosis in fetal diaphragmatic hernia. Am J Obstet Gynecol 1992;166:9-13.

Smythe JF, Copel JA, Kleinman CS. Outcome of prenatally detected cardiac malformations. Am J Cardiol 1992;69:1471-4.

Snijders RJM, Sherrod C, Gosden CM, Nicolaides KH. Fetal growth retardation: associated malformations and chromosomal abnormalities. Am J Obstet Gynecol 1993;168:547-55.

Snijders RJM, Shawwa L, Nicolaides KH. Fetal choroid plexus cysts and trisomy 18: assessment of risk based on ultrasound findings and maternal age. Prenat Diagn 1994; 14: 1119-27.

Stoll C, Alembik Y, Roth MP, Dott B, Sauvage P. Risk factors in internal urinary system malformations. Pediatr Nephrol 1990;4:319-23.

Tannirandorn Y, Nicolini U, Nicolaidis P, Fisk NM, Arulkumaran S, Rodeck CH. Fetal cystic hygromata: insights gained from fetal blood sampling. Prenat Diagn 1990;10:189-93.

Thelander HE, Pryor HB. Abnormal patterns of growth and development in mongolism. An anthropometric study. Clin Pediatr 1966;5:493.

Thorpe-Beeston G, Gosden CM, Nicolaides KH. Congenital diaphragmatic hernia: associated malformations and chromosomal defects. Fetal Ther 1989;4:21-8.

Thorpe-Beeston JG, Gosden CM, Nicolaides KH. Choroid plexus cysts and chromosomal defects. Br J Radiol 1990;63:783-6.

Toi A, Simpson GF, Filly RA. Ultrasonically evident fetal nuchal skin thickening: is it specific for Down syndrome? Am J Obstet Gynecol 1987;156:150-3.

Touloukian RJ. Intestinal atresia. Clin Perinatol 1978;5:3-18.

Turner GM, Twining P. The facial profile in the diagnosis of fetal abnormalities. Clin Radiol 1993;47:389-95.

Twining P, Whalley DR, Lewin E, Foulkes K. Is a short femur length a useful ultrasound marker for Down's Syndrome? Br J Radiol 1991a;64:990-2.

Twining P, Zuccollo J, Clewes J, Swallow J. Fetal choroid plexus cysts: a prospective study and review of the literature. Br J Radiol 1991b;64:98-102.

Twining P. Echogenic foci in the fetal heart: incidence and association with chromosomal disease. Ultrasound Obstet Gynecol 1993,3(Suppl. 2):Abstract 190.

Van de Geijn EJ, van Vugt, Sollie JE, van Geijn HP. Ultrasonographic diagnosis and perinatal management of fetal abdominal wall defects. Fetal Diagn Ther 1991;6:2-10.

Van Zalen-Spock MM, Van Vugt JMG, Karsdorp VHM, Maas R, Van Geijn HP. Ultrasound diagnosis of fetal abnormalities and cytogenetic evaluation. Prenat Diagn 1991;11:655-60.

Vergani P, Ghidini A, Strobelt N, Locatelli A, Mariani S, Bertalero C, Cavallone M. Prognostic indicators in the prenatal diagnosis of agenesis of corpus callosum. Am J Obstet Gynecol 1994;170:753-8.

Ville Y, Borghi E, Pons JC, Lelorc'h M. Fetal karyotype from cystic hygroma fluid. Prenat Diagn 1992;12:139-43.

Vintzileos AM, Campbell WA, Weinbaum PJ, Nochimson DJ. Perinatal management and outcome of fetal ventriculomegaly. Obstet Gynecol 1987;69: 5-11.

Wald NJ, Cuckle NS, Densem JW, *et al.* Maternal serum screening for Down's syndrome in early pregnancy. Br Med J 1988;276:883-7.

Walkinshaw S, Pilling D, Spriggs A. Isolated choroid plexus cysts - the need for routine offer of karyotyping. Prenat Diagn 1994;14:663-7.

Watson WJ, Katz VL, Chescheir NC, Miller RC, Menard MK, Hansen WF. The cisterna magna in second-trimester fetuses with abnormal karyotypes. Obstet Gynecol 1992;79:723-5.

Watson WJ, Miller RC, Menard MK, Chescheir NC, Katz VL, Hansen WF, Wolf EJ. Ultrasonographic measurement of fetal nuchal skin to screen for chromosomal abnormalities. Am J Obstet Gynecol 1994;170:583-6.

Wilson RD, Chitayat D, McGillivray BC. Fetal ultrasound abnormalities: correlation with fetal karyotype, autopsy findings, and postnatal outcome - five-year prospective study. Am J Med Genet 1992;44:586-90.

Winston YE, Horger III EO. Down syndrome and femur length. Am J Obstet Gynecol 1988;159:1810.

Zerres K, Schuler H, Gembruch U, Bald R, Hansmann M, Schwanitz G. Chromosomal findings in fetuses with prenatally diagnosed cysts of the choroid plexus. Hum Genet 1992;89:301-4.

Assessment of risks

OVERVIEW

Ultrasound studies have demonstrated that major chromosomal defects are often associated with multiple fetal abnormalities (see Chapter 1). Conversely, in fetuses with multiple abnormalities the frequency of chromosomal defects is high and in most cases fetal karyotyping is offered irrespective of maternal age.

For apparently isolated abnormalities, there are large differences in the reported prevalence of associated chromosomal defects and it is uncertain whether in such cases karyotyping should be undertaken, especially for those abnormalities that have a high prevalence in the general population and for which the prognosis in the absence of a chromosomal defect is good.

Since the frequency of chromosomal defects is associated with maternal age, it is possible that the wide range of results reported in the various studies is the mere consequence of differences in the maternal age distribution of the populations examined. In addition, since chromosomal abnormalities are associated with a high rate of intrauterine death, differences may arise from the fact that studies were undertaken at different stages of pregnancy. Therefore, we propose that, in the calculation of risks for chromosomal defects, it is necessary to take into account ultrasound findings as well as the maternal age and the gestational age at the time of the scan.

Traditionally, counselling parents as to the risk of fetal chromosomal defects has depended on the provision of live birth incidences of trisomy 21. However, with ultrasound screening it is necessary to establish prevalences for all chromosomal defects that are associated with anatomical and biometrical abnormalities.

Additionally, since the various chromosomal defects differ in their rate of intrauterine lethality, it is necessary to establish maternal and gestational age-specific risks for each of these chromosomal defects. For example, exomphalos is associated with trisomy 18 but the risk for this chromosomal defect increases with maternal age and decreases with gestation; the prevalence of trisomy 18 in the presence of exomphalos is lower if the maternal age is 20 years rather than 40 years and it is higher if the gestation is 12 weeks rather than 24 weeks. Similarly, to determine whether apparently isolated choroid plexus cysts at 20 weeks of gestation are associated with an increased risk for trisomy 18, it is essential to know the prevalence of trisomy 18 at 20 weeks, based on the maternal age distribution of the population that is examined.

ASSOCIATION WITH MATERNAL AGE AND GESTATION

Trisomy 21

Langdon Down first described the syndrome in 1866 and noted that the *'skin is deficient in elasticity, giving the appearance of being too large for the body'*.

Fraser and Mitchell (1876) noted a lack of hereditary factors but an association with advanced maternal age. Subsequently, Shuttleworth (1909), in a study of 350 cases, reported that a considerable proportion of affected infants, *'from one-half to one-third, were born to women approaching the climacteric'*.

The trisomic origin of the syndrome was first described by Bleyer (1934), who proposed an association with degeneration of the ovum. Antonarakis (1991) examined DNA polymorphisms in Down syndrome infants and demonstrated that 95% of non-dysjunction trisomy 21 is maternal in origin.

Prevalence in live births

In the late 1970s and 1980s, at the time of the introduction of prenatal diagnosis, eight large surveys were carried out to assess the age-specific prevalence of trisomy 21 in live births (Hook & Chambers 1977, Hook & Fabia 1978, Hook & Lindsjo 1978, Trimble & Baird 1978, Sutherland *et al* 1979, Koulischer & Gillerot 1980, Young *et al* 1980, Huether *et al* 1981).

In most studies the observed frequencies were adjusted to correct for under-ascertainment, lack of information on the maternal age distribution or the effect of selective abortion after prenatal diagnosis. For example, studies of trisomy 21 infants have demonstrated that in 50–70% of cases the condition is not entered on the birth certificate; therefore, the number of cases with trisomy 21 reported in surveys where information was obtained from birth certificates was multiplied by a factor of 2–3.

Some surveys provided data on the number of cases with trisomy 21 for each year of maternal age but information on the total number of births was available only for 5-year intervals; in these surveys estimates of the number of births for each year of maternal age were derived from distributions observed in populations where year-by-year data were available.

There are only two surveys with almost complete ascertainment; in a survey in South Belgium every neonate was examined for features of trisomy 21 (Koulischer and Gillerot 1980) and in a survey in Sweden information was verified using several sources such as hospital notes, cytogenetic laboratories, genetic clinics and schools for mentally handicapped (Hook & Lindsjo 1978).

Cuckle *et al* (1987) combined the data from all eight surveys on a total of 3,289,114 births to determine the prevalence of trisomy 21 at each maternal age; regression analysis was applied to smooth out fluctuations in the observed rates (Figure 2.1). Hecht and Hook (1994) used only the data from the two surveys with almost complete ascertainment and calculated maternal age-specific frequencies with 90% confidence intervals (Figure 2.1). The results of the two studies were similar and the estimated risk for trisomy 21 increased exponentially with maternal age.

Prevalence during pregnancy

In the 1970s, genetic amniocentesis at 16–20 weeks of gestation was offered to women aged 35 years or older because they were considered to be at high risk for trisomy 21. In the 1980s, chorionic villus sampling and early amniocentesis were introduced for fetal karyotyping at 9–14 weeks of gestation.

Data from prenatal studies confirmed that the prevalence of trisomy 21 increases with maternal age but they also showed that the prevalence during pregnancy is higher than at birth.

The combined data from two multicentre studies of amniocentesis at 16–20 weeks of gestation, one in the USA involving 56,094 pregnancies and another of 52,965 cases in Europe, showed that at 16–20 weeks the prevalence of trisomy 21 is approximately 30% higher than at birth (Table 2.1; Ferguson-Smith and Yates 1984, Hook *et al* 1984).

Data from fetal karyotyping at 9–14 weeks in 15,793 cases showed that the prevalence of trisomy 21 is 50% higher than at birth (Table 2.1, Snijders *et al* 1995a).

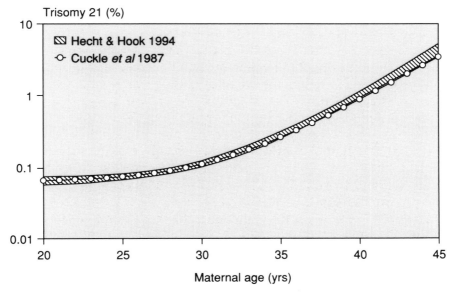

Figure 2.1 Prevalence of trisomy 21 in live births as estimated by Cuckle *et al* (1987; prevalence of trisomy 21 = 0.000627 + $e^{-16.2395+0.286 \times age}$) and Hecht & Hook (1994; prevalence of trisomy 21 = 0.000631 + $e^{-16.60785+0.2994 \times age}$); the 90% confidence interval in the latter is indicated by the shaded area.

Table 2.1 Prevalence of trisomy 21 in live births, at 16–20 weeks of gestation and at 9–14 weeks in women aged 35 years or more.

Author	Group	N	Trisomy 21
Hecht & Hook 1994	Live births	281,613	0.68%
Hook *et al* 1984,	16-20 weeks	108,569	0.97%
Ferguson-Smith & Yates 1984			
Snijders *et al* 1995	9-14 weeks	15,793	1.34%

Data from the subgroup of women aged 35–42 years were used to examine the slopes of the regression lines describing the relationship between maternal age and prevalence of trisomy 21. The almost parallel increase of frequencies suggests that there are no maternal age-related differences in the rate of intrauterine lethality for trisomy 21 (Figure 2.2). It can therefore be assumed that the ratio of the prevalence observed at a given gestation compared to the prevalence at birth is similar for women of all ages.

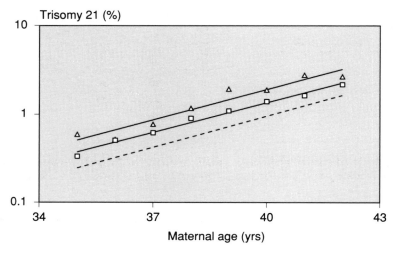

Figure 2.2 Prevalence of trisomy 21 with maternal age at 11 weeks of gestation (Δ), at 17 weeks (□) and in live births (----). The slopes of the regression lines are similar, suggesting that in trisomy 21 the rate of intrauterine lethality is similar in all maternal age groups.

If the prevalence of trisomy 21 in live births is 1.0, then the relative prevalence at 17 weeks of gestation is 1.4 and at 11 weeks is 1.8. Using these three points, estimates for the relative prevalence at different gestations were derived (Figure 2.3).

Maternal and gestational age-specific risks for trisomy 21 were then calculated by multiplying the maternal age-specific prevalences in live births with the relative prevalence at a given gestation (Table 2.2).

Gestation	Relative prevalence
Live births	1.00
35 wks	1.04
30 wks	1.10
25 wks	1.18
20 wks	1.30
18 wks	1.37
16 wks	1.45
14 wks	1.56
12 wks	1.70
10 wks	1.90

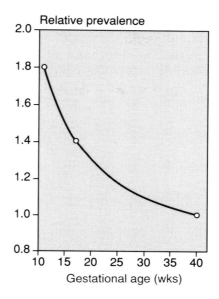

Figure 2.3 Estimated relative prevalence of trisomy 21 at different gestations compared to the prevalence in live births which was considered to be 1.0.

Table 2.2 Estimated risk for trisomy 21 (1/number given in the table) in relation to maternal age and gestation. The full table is given in Appendix 2.

Age (yrs)	Gestation (wks)									
	10	12	14	16	18	20	25	30	35	Birth
20	804	898	981	1053	1117	1175	1294	1388	1464	1527
25	712	795	868	933	989	1040	1146	1229	1297	1352
30	471	526	575	617	655	688	758	813	858	895
35	187	210	229	246	261	274	302	324	342	356
40	51	57	62	67	71	74	82	88	93	97

Trisomy 18

Trisomy 18, first described by Edwards (1960), is the second most frequent trisomy at birth with a prevalence of 0.16 per 1,000 live births (Hook *et al* 1979).

In trisomy 18, unlike trisomy 21, there are no available data on the maternal age-specific risks in live births. However, data from women aged ≥35 years undergoing first or second trimester fetal karyotyping have demonstrated that the prevalence of trisomy 18 increases with maternal age (Figure 2.4; Ferguson-Smith & Yates 1984, Hook *et al* 1984, Snijders *et al* 1995a).

The slope of the increase in trisomy 18 with maternal age in the prenatal studies was not substantially different from that of trisomy 21 in live births. These findings suggest that, as with trisomy 21, there are no maternal age-related differences in the rate of intrauterine lethality for trisomy 18.

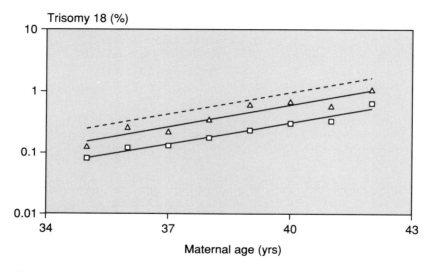

Figure 2.4 The prevalence of trisomy 18 at 9–14 weeks of gestation (△) and the prevalence of trisomy 18 at 16–20 weeks (□) compared to the prevalence of trisomy 21 in live births (----) in women aged 35–42 years.

Compared to the prevalence of trisomy 21 in live births, which was considered to be 1.0, the prevalences of trisomy 18 in live births and at 17 and 11 weeks of gestation are 0.09, 0.34 and 0.71, respectively. Using regression analysis on these three points, estimates for the relative prevalence of trisomy 18 at different gestations were derived (Figure 2.5).

Estimates of maternal and gestational age-specific risks for trisomy 18 were obtained by multiplying the maternal age-specific prevalences of trisomy 21 in live births with the estimated relative prevalence of trisomy 18 at a given gestation (Table 2.3). For example, in a 35 year old woman, where the prevalence of trisomy 21 in live births is 1/356, the birth prevalence of trisomy 18 is 0.0848 x 1/356.18 or 1/4,202; at 20 weeks it is 0.3119 x 1/356.18 or 1/1,142 and at 10 weeks it is 0.7660 x 1/356.18 or 1/465.

Gestation	Relative prevalence
Live births	0.0848
35 wks	0.1172
30 wks	0.1604
25 wks	0.2210
20 wks	0.3119
18 wks	0.3623
16 wks	0.4255
14 wks	0.5067
12 wks	0.6141
10 wks	0.7660

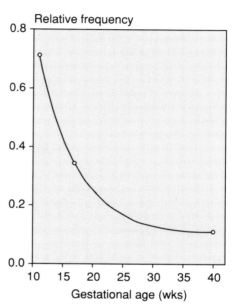

Figure 2.5 Estimated relative prevalence of trisomy 18 at different gestations, compared to a value of 1.0 for the prevalence of trisomy 21 in live births.

Table 2.3. Estimated risk for trisomy 18 (1/number given in the table) in relation to maternal age and gestation. The full table is given in Appendix 2.

Age (yrs)	Gestation (wks)									
	10	12	14	16	18	20	25	30	35	Birth
20	1993	2484	3015	3590	4215	4897	6909	9516	13028	18013
25	1765	2200	2670	3179	3732	4336	6118	8427	11536	15951
30	1168	1456	1766	2103	2469	2869	4048	5575	7633	10554
35	465	580	703	837	983	1142	1612	2220	3039	4202
40	126	157	191	227	267	310	437	602	824	1139

Trisomy 13

Trisomy 13, first described by Patau *et al* (1960), is the third most frequent trisomy at birth with a prevalence of 0.083 per 1,000 live births (Hook 1980).

As with trisomy 18, there are no data on the maternal age-specific risks in live births, but data from women aged $\geq$35 years undergoing first or second trimester fetal karyotyping have reported that the prevalence of trisomy 13 increases with maternal age (Snijders *et al* 1994b). As with trisomies 21 and 18, the slope of the increase in trisomy 13 with maternal age in the prenatal studies was not substantially different from that of trisomy 21 in live births (Figure 2.6).

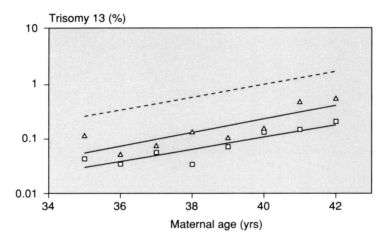

Figure 2.6 The prevalence of trisomy 13 at 9–14 weeks of gestation ($\triangle$) and the prevalence of trisomy 13 at 16–20 weeks ($\square$) compared to the prevalence of trisomy 21 in live births (----) in women aged 35–42 years.

If the prevalence of trisomy 21 in live births is 1.0, then the prevalences of trisomy 13 in live births and at 17 and 11 weeks of gestation are 0.04, 0.13 and 0.22, respectively. The risks for trisomy 13 for each maternal age and each gestational age were estimated from the maternal age-specific incidence of trisomy 21 in live births and the estimated relative prevalence of trisomy 13 at different gestations (Figure 2.7, Table 2.4). For example, in women aged 35 years, where the birth incidence of trisomy 21 is 1/356, the estimated incidence of trisomy 13 at birth is 0.036 x 1/356.18 or 1/9,896.

Gestation	Relative prevalence
Live births	0.0360
35 wks	0.0457
30 wks	0.0587
25 wks	0.0770
20 wks	0.1042
18 wks	0.1193
16 wks	0.1383
14 wks	0.1626
12 wks	0.1951
10 wks	0.2405

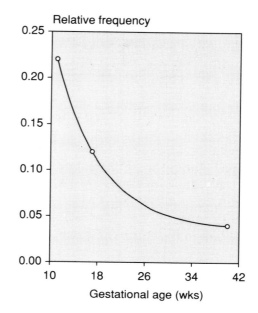

Figure 2.7 Estimated relative prevalence of trisomy 13 at different gestations, compared to a value of 1.0 for the prevalence of trisomy 21 in live births.

Table 2.4 Estimated risk for trisomy 13 (1/number given in the table) in relation to maternal age and gestation. The full table is given Appendix 2.

Age (yrs)	Gestation (wks)									
	10	12	14	16	18	20	25	30	35	Birth
20	6347	7826	9389	11042	12795	14656	19854	26002	33387	42423
25	5621	6930	8314	9778	11330	12978	17581	23026	29565	37567
30	3719	4585	5501	6470	7496	8587	11632	15234	19561	24856
35	1481	1826	2190	2576	2985	3419	4631	6065	7788	9896
40	401	495	594	698	809	927	1255	1644	2111	2683

Turner syndrome

In live births, the prevalence of Turner syndrome is 0.024% (Hsu *et al* 1992) and the condition is not associated with increased postnatal mortality. However, the relatively high frequency of Turner syndrome observed in spontaneous abortuses and at prenatal diagnosis (Carr 1963, Schreinemachers *et al* 1982,

Ferguson-Smith and Yates 1984, Snijders *et al* 1995a) indicates that the syndrome may have different phenotypes, some of which are associated with a high lethality at an early stage of pregnancy. Turner syndrome is usually due to loss of the paternal X chromosome and consequently the frequency of conception of 45,X embryos, unlike that of trisomies, is unrelated to maternal age (Table 2.5, Figure 2.8).

Table 2.5 Prevalence of Turner syndrome found at antenatal karyotyping at 9–14 weeks of gestation and at 16–20 weeks.

Age	9-14 weeks		16-20 weeks	
	N	**Turner synd**	**N**	**Turner synd**
35-36	5439	7 (0.129%)	19,567	10 (0.051%)
37-38	5066	5 (0.099%)	21,119	10 (0.047%)
39-40	3331	0	18,213	6 (0.033%)
41-45	1957	3 (0.153%)	22,709	1 (0.004%)
Total	**15,793**	**15 (0.095%)**	**72,234**	**27 (0.037%)**

Gestation	Prevalence
Live births	1/4200
35 wks	1/4000
30 wks	1/3800
25 wks	1/3500
20 wks	1/3000
15 wks	1/2000
10 wks	1/1000

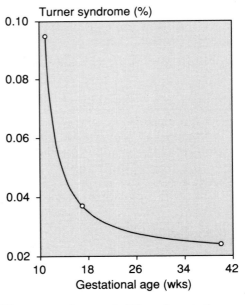

Figure 2.8 Estimated prevalence of Turner syndrome at different gestations.

Other sex chromosome defects

The main sex chromosome defects, other than Turner syndrome, are 47,XXX, 47,XXY and 47,XYY. In infants with 47,XYY, physical appearance, mental development and fertility are normal. However, compared to normal infants, they have an increased incidence of mild impairments in language and reading, hyperactivity, impulsivity and a tendency for more aggressive behaviour. In both Klinefelter syndrome (47,XXY) and in 47,XXX females, mental retardation is unlikely and, although intelligence tends to be less than that of siblings, there is a large individual variation. Adults tend to be tall but their head circumference is generally reduced. In 47,XXX, fertility is usually normal, whereas 47,XXY individuals are infertile. In 47,XXY, minor congenital abnormalities, most frequently clinodactyly, are found in about one fourth of neonates. Adults with 47,XXY have increased susceptibility to autoimmune disease, malignancy, and cerebrovascular disease.

In live births, these sex chromosome aneuploidies are more common than trisomies; in a total of 68,159 live births (for all maternal ages) the prevalence was 0.17% compared to 0.14% for the trisomies (Table 2.6; Hsu *et al* 1992). In prenatal series, however, which are confined to women aged ≥35 years, the prevalence of trisomies was higher (Table 2.6).

Table 2.6 Prevalence of sex chromosome aneuploidies other than Turner syndrome and prevalence of autosomal trisomies in live births (Hsu *et al* 1992), and in first and second trimester prenatal studies (Schreinemachers *et al* 1982, Ferguson Smith & Yates 1984, Snijders *et al* 1994a).

Chromosomal defect	Live births (all ages) n=68,159	16-20 weeks (35-42 years) n=68,273	9-14 weeks (35-42 years) n=15,280
Sex chromosomes	0.172%	0.266%	0.085%
47,XYY	0.066%	0.038%	0.013%
47,XXY	0.066%	0.129%	0.039%
47,XXX	0.040%	0.099%	0.033%
Autosomal trisomies	0.137%	1.157%	1.912%
47,+21	0.120%	0.879%	1.336%
47,+18	0.013%	0.205%	0.424%
47,+13	0.004%	0.073%	0.152%

These findings suggest that sex chromosome defects are associated with a much lower intrauterine lethality than trisomies and/or that the association with maternal age is less pronounced.

There is no obvious explanation for the observation that the frequencies of 47,XXX, 47,XXY and 47,XYY at 9–14 weeks of gestation were much lower than at 16–20 weeks.

A follow up study of pregnancies with sex chromosome defects diagnosed at second trimester amniocentesis, and where the parents chose to continue with the pregnancy, confirmed that the rate of intrauterine lethality is low; in a total of 106 singleton pregnancies with 47,XXX (n=39), 47,XXY (n=35), or 47,XYY (n=32) the rate of fetal loss was only 1.9% (two cases), which is similar to the 1.7% loss rate in normal pregnancies after second trimester amniocentesis (Hook 1983, Tabor *et al* 1986).

Data from women aged 35–42 years undergoing second trimester fetal karyotyping indicate that the prevalences of 47,XXX and 47,XXY increase with maternal age but the slope of increase is much less pronounced than that for trisomies, while there is a tendency for the prevalence of 47,XYY to decrease (Figure 2.9; Schreinemachers *et al* 1982, Ferguson-Smith & Yates 1984).

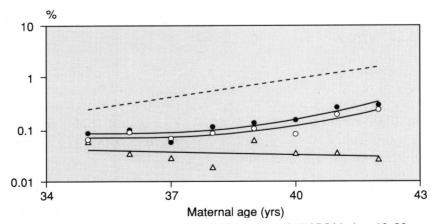

Figure 2.9 Prevalence of 47,XXY (●), 47,XXX (○) and 47,XYY (△) at 16–20 weeks compared to trisomy 21 in live births (----) in women aged 35–42 years.

Since the rate of intrauterine lethality of these chromosomal defects is not higher than in chromosomally normal fetuses, it can be assumed that the prevalence does not change with gestation. Table 2.7 provides estimates for prevalences with maternal age that were derived by combining information from the overall prevalence in live births and data from the amniocentesis studies (Table 2.7).

Table 2.7 Estimated risk for 47,XXX, 47,XXY and 47,XYY (1/number given in the table) in relation to maternal age. Given the low intrauterine lethality, it was assumed that prevalences remain the same throughout pregnancy.

Maternal age	Prevalence of chromosomal defects		
(yrs)	47,XXX	47,XXY	47,XYY
<35	1400	1200	2250
35-37	1400	1200	2500
38-40	1100	900	2750
>40	650	500	3000

Triploidy

Polyploidy, caused by fertilisation with multiple sperm or by failure of cell cleavage in the first mitotic division of the fertilised egg, affects about 2% of recognised conceptions (Boyers *et al* 1987). Triploidy is highly lethal and it is very rarely observed in live births. At 9–14 weeks of gestation the prevalence is only 0.05% (Snijders *et al* 1995a) and at 16–20 weeks the prevalence is 0.002% (Ferguson-Smith *et al* 1984).

The prevalence of triploidy is not related to maternal age, but is strongly related to gestational age because of the very high rate of intrauterine lethality. On the assumption that the prevalence at six weeks of gestation is 2%, at 11 weeks is 0.05% and at 40 weeks is 0%, it was possible to estimate the prevalence of triploidy throughout pregnancy (Figure 2.10).

Ultrasonographically, there are two phenotypic expressions of triploidy. The first is characterised by a molar placenta and this is highly lethal during the first 20 weeks of pregnancy because it is rarely seen after this gestation. In the second type, the placenta appears normal but the fetus presents with severe asymmetrical intrauterine growth retardation at 20–28 weeks.

Gestation	Prevalence
20 wks	1/250000
18 wks	1/100000
16 wks	1/ 30000
14 wks	1/ 10000
12 wks	1/ 3500
10 wks	1/ 1000
8 wks	1/ 350
6 wks	1/ 50

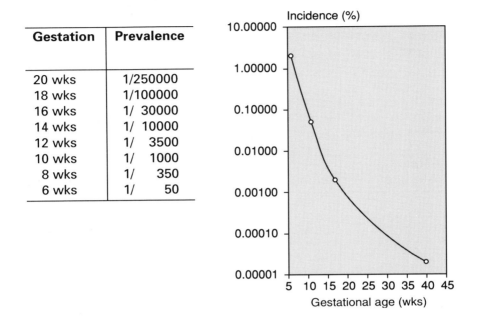

Figure 2.10 Estimated prevalence of triploidy at different gestations.

Intrauterine lethality of chromosomal defects

The rate of intrauterine lethality of the various chromosomal defects can be calculated from the differences between the incidences at first and second trimester karyotyping and incidences in live births (Table 2.8).

For trisomy 21, if the prevalence at birth is 1.00, the relative prevalence at 16 weeks of gestation is 1.45 (see Figure 2.3), and the rate of intrauterine lethality between 16 weeks and birth is 28%. This is similar to the 30% rate observed by Hook *et al* (1983) in pregnancies where a chromosomal defect was diagnosed at second trimester amniocentesis and the parents decided against termination (Table 2.8).

For trisomy 18, the estimated rate of intrauterine lethality between 16 weeks and birth (71%) was also similar to the 68% observed by Hook *et al* (1983). However, for trisomy 13 the estimated rate was higher, while for Turner syndrome it was lower than that observed by Hook *et al* (1983). For both chromosomal defects, the estimated rates may be more accurate than the observed ones, because the number of cases that were examined is very small (four cases of trisomy 13 and 11 of Turner syndrome).

Table 2.8 Estimates for spontaneous loss rates of fetuses with various chromosomal defects on the basis of prevalences at first and second trimester karyotyping and in live births. The last column reports the frequency of spontaneous fetal death for chromosomal defects diagnosed by mid-trimester amniocentesis (Hook *et al* 1983).

Chromosomal defect	Estimated loss rate		Observed loss rate
	10 wks - birth	16 wks - birth	16 wks - birth
Trisomy 21	47%	31%	30%
Trisomy 18	86%	74%	68%
Trisomy 13	83%	71%	43%
Turner syndrome	76%	52%	75%
47,XXX	~5%	~3%	0%
47,XXY	~5%	~3%	1%
47,XYY	~5%	~3%	3%
Triploidy	>99%	>99%	100%

Ultrasound findings, maternal age and gestation

A study of fetuses that were karyotyped because ultrasound examination had revealed at least one abnormality and/or growth retardation demonstrated that the frequency of autosomal aneuploidies increased with maternal age, whereas for Turner syndrome and triploidy there was a tendency for a decrease in prevalence with age (Table 2.9; Nicolaides *et al* 1992a).

The most likely explanation for these findings is that the frequencies of Turner syndrome and triploid conceptions are similar for all age groups, but younger women are more able to sustain pregnancies with these highly lethal abnormalities into the second and third trimesters of pregnancy.

Table 2.9 Frequency of chromosomal defects in relation to maternal age in a series of 2,086 fetuses with ultrasonographically detectable abnormalities and/or growth retardation (Nicolaides *et al* 1992a).

Maternal age	Chromosomal defects			
	Total	Trisomies	Turner	Triploidy
15-24 years	10%	4.8%	1.5%	1.9%
25-34 years	14%	7.3%	2.0%	2.4%
35-44 years	26%	22.2%	1.6%	0.7%

This study has also demonstrated that, in the assessment of risk for chromosomal defects, not only maternal age but also gestation should be considered. Thus, the pattern of chromosomal defects as well as the prevalence differed depending on gestation; the overall prevalence decreased with gestation and both Turner syndrome and triploidy, which are highly lethal, were not seen during the third trimester (Table 2.10).

Table 2.10 Prevalence of chromosomal defects in relation to gestational age in a series of 2,086 fetuses with ultrasonographically detectable abnormalities and/or growth retardation (Nicolaides *et al* 1992a).

Gestational age	Chromosomal defects			
	Total	Trisomies	Turner	Triploidy
15-23 wks	17%	9.5%	3.3%	2.7%
24-31 wks	11%	7.2%	0.2%	2.0%
32-39 wks	12%	8.9%	0.0%	0.0%

ASSOCIATION WITH FETAL STRUCTURAL ABNORMALITIES

Presence or absence of multiple abnormalities

As demonstrated in Chapter 1, the frequency of chromosomal defects associated with each abnormality is much higher when there are multiple rather than apparently isolated abnormalities; these findings are summarised in Table 2.11.

For apparently isolated abnormalities, there may be only a minor increase in the maternal and gestational age-related prevalence of a given chromosomal defect. The overall frequency of chromosomal defects for apparently isolated abnormalities is less than 1%, irrespective of whether the defect is major, such as exomphalos, or minor, such as choroid plexus cysts. However, the sonographer should be aware of the phenotypic expression of the various chromosomal defects and specifically search for all potential abnormalities before arriving at the conclusion that a given abnormality is apparently isolated. It is possible that, in those studies reporting a high frequency of chromosomal defects for apparently isolated abnormalities, the sonographers did not undertake a thorough examination of all other fetal parts or the quality of the ultrasound equipment used was inadequate.

Table 2.11 Summary of findings from different studies (see Chapter 1) that examined the prevalence of fetal chromosomal defects in fetuses with isolated and multiple sonographically detected abnormalities.

Abnormality	N	Isolated	Multiple
Ventriculomegaly	690	2%	17%
Holoprosencephaly	94	4%	39%
Choroid plexus cysts	1884	1%	48%
Posterior fossa cyst	101	0%	52%
Facial cleft	118	0%	51%
Micrognathia	65	-	62%
Cystic hygromata	312	52%	71%
Nuchal oedema	371	19%	45%
Diaphragmatic hernia	173	2%	49%
Heart defects	829	16%	66%
Duodenal atresia	44	38%	64%
Echogenic bowel	196	7%	42%
Exomphalos	495	8%	46%
Renal abnormalities	1780	3%	24%
Talipes	127	0%	?33%
Small for gestational age	621	4%	38%

In some cases, even for apparently isolated abnormalities, the frequency of chromosomal defects is high. An example of this is cystic hygromata, and the most likely explanation for this is that, in many cases of Turner syndrome, the associated cardiac abnormalities are not easily detectable by ultrasonography. For other abnormalities, such as nuchal oedema and duodenal atresia, the most common chromosomal defect is trisomy 21, where associated abnormalities are often subtle and may not be detected by ultrasonography.

Sonographic scoring system I

The overall risk for chromosomal defects increases with the total number of abnormalities that are identified. In a study of 2,086 fetuses that were karyotyped because ultrasound examination had revealed at least one fetal abnormality and/or growth retardation, the frequency of chromosomal defects increased with the number of abnormalities (Table 2.12; Nicolaides *et al* 1992a). It is therefore recommended that, when an abnormality/marker is detected at routine ultrasound examination, a thorough check is made for the other features of the chromosomal defect(s) known to be associated with that marker; should additional abnormalities be identified the risk is dramatically increased.

Table 2.12 Prevalence of chromosomal defects in relation to number of sonographically detected abnormalities (Nicolaides *et al* 1992a).

Abnormalities	N	Chromosomal defects
1	1128	2%
2	490	11%
3	220	32%
4	115	52%
5	53	66%
6	40	63%
7	16	69%
≥ 8	24	92%

Sonographic scoring system II

Benacerraf *et al* (1994) proposed a scoring system for the risk of trisomies according to the presence or absence of anatomic abnormalities, such as cardiac defect or hydrocephalus, thickened nuchal fold, short femur, short humerus, mild hydronephrosis or pyelectasia, choroid plexus cysts, and hyperechogenic bowel (Table 2.13).

In a study of 60 fetuses with trisomy 21 (n=45), trisomy 18 (n=13) or trisomy 13 (n=2), and 106 normal controls, a sonographic score of ≥ 2 identified 73% of fetuses with trisomy 21, 85% of those with trisomy 18 and both fetuses with trisomy 13; the false positive rate was 4% (Benacerraf *et al* 1994).

In an expanded series of 97 trisomic and 694 normal control fetuses, a score of ≥ 1 identified 86% of the trisomic fetuses and the false positive rate was 13% (Benacerraf *et al* 1994). Furthermore, the data of this study suggested that a score of zero may be associated with a three-fold reduction in the maternal age-related risk for trisomies.

Table 2.13 Scoring system for the assessment of risk for trisomies based on the presence or absence of specific abnormalities.

Feature	Score
Anatomic abnormality	2
Thickened nuchal fold	2
Short femur	1
Short humerus	1
Pyelectasia	1
Choroid plexus cysts	1
Echogenic bowel	1
Total	**9**

THE EXAMPLE OF CHOROID PLEXUS CYSTS AND TRISOMY 18

This example illustrates how data from observational and screening studies can be combined to derive risks for chromosomal defects, taking into account maternal age, gestation and the presence or absence of additional abnormalities.

Fetal choroid plexus cysts (CPCs) are potentially useful markers for trisomy 18 in as much as they are present in about 50% of affected fetuses and they are easily seen in the standard biparietal diameter view which is obtained for all routine ultrasound scans. However, practising sonographers receive contradictory advice as to whether karyotyping should be offered to all women (1–2% of the pregnant population) where fetal CPCs are diagnosed.

During the last decade several prenatal studies have been performed and the accumulated data allow development of a model for comprehensive assessment of risks. Tables derived in this section will need validation and further study but they provide at least some guidelines for counselling parents.

To calculate the risks for trisomy 18 in mid-trimester fetuses with CPCs it is essential to know: (i) the prevalence of trisomy 18 at mid-gestation, (ii) the prevalence of CPCs at mid-gestation, (iii) the prevalence of CPCs in fetuses with trisomy 18, (iv) the incidence of additional abnormalities in fetuses with CPCs.

Prevalence of trisomy 18 at mid-gestation

The maternal age-specific risks for trisomy 18 at 20 weeks of gestation are given in Table 2.3. The risk increases from 1/4,897 in a 20 year old to 1/1,142 in a women aged 35 years and 1/98 in a woman aged 44 years.

Prevalence of choroid plexus cysts at mid-gestation

There are 13 population screening studies that provide data on the prevalence of CPCs (Table 2.14).

Table 2.14 Screening studies on the prevalence of choroid plexus cysts providing data on gestational age (GA), diameter of the cysts and the prevalence of trisomy 18 in those with apparently isolated cysts and those with multiple abnormalities. The top seven studies were on referred populations but those referred because of choroid plexus cysts were excluded and the bottom six studies were unselected population based studies.

Author	GA (wk)	N	Prevalence	Size (mm)	Isolated	Multiple
Chitkara et al 88	16-42	6,288	41 (0.65%)	≥3	-/38	1/3
Clark et al 88	16-22	2,820	5 (0.18%)	≥3	-/5	-
DeRoo et al 88	14-21	2,084	17 (0.81%)	>2	-/17	-
Chan et al 89	15-24	513	13 (2.53%)	≥3	-/13	-
Platt et al 91	15-22	7,350	71 (0.96%)	?	-/67	3/4
Perpignano et al 92	14-33	3,769	87 (2.31%)	≥2	3/86	1/1
Porto et al 93	15-22	3,247	63 (1.94%)	≥2	-/59	3/4
Ostlere et al 90	16-18	11,700	100 (0.85%)	≥2	-/96	3/4
Achiron et al 91	18-22	5,400	30 (0.56%)	?	1/29	1/1
Chinn et al 91	18-24	1,045	38 (3.64%)	≥2	-/36	- /2
Twining et al 91	18-20	4,541	19 (0.42%)	≥3	-/16	2/3
Howard et al 92	18-20	4,765	51 (1.07%)	?	1/51	-
Walkinshaw et al 94	17-19	15,565	152 (0.98%)	?	3/140	- /12
Total	**14-42**	**69,087**	**687 (0.99%)**		**8/613**	**14/34**

Six papers reported on routine scanning of populations at 16–24 weeks and seven papers reported findings in referred populations but excluding referrals for CPCs.

In those studies that diagnosed CPCs with a minimum diameter of 2mm rather than 3mm, the prevalence tended to be higher. In addition, the prevalence for the 2mm CPCs was higher in the more recent studies, presumably reflecting improved resolution in ultrasound equipment. In two studies the upper gestational age of the fetuses was more than 24 weeks and the prevalence would have been underestimated because CPCs usually resolve after this gestation.

Despite these limitations, it could be assumed that the mean prevalence of CPCs is 1.0%.

Prevalence of choroid plexus cysts in trisomy 18

In three studies reporting on the phenotypic expression of trisomy 18, the mean prevalence of choroid plexus cysts was about 50% (Table 2.15).

Table 2.15 Prevalence of choroid plexus cysts (CPCs) in fetuses with trisomy 18 at 15–25 weeks of gestation.

Author	Study period	Gestation (wks)	Total	CPCs
Benacerraf et al 90a	1983-89	15-19	17	5 (29%)
Nyberg et al 93a	1984-92	15-24	27	10 (37%)
Snijders et al 94	1987-93	16-23	58	38 (66%)
Total	1983-93	15-24	102	53 (53%)

The large differences between the studies may be the consequence of the relatively small number of cases in each study, differences in the referred populations and under-diagnosis of CPCs in the studies of Benacerraf et al (1990a) and Nyberg et al (1993a). These two studies included cases from the early 1980s; prenatal diagnosis of CPCs was first reported in 1984 (Chudleigh et al 1984), and it was not until 1986 that the possibility of an association with trisomy 18 was raised (Nicolaides et al 1986).

Additional abnormalities in fetuses with choroid plexus cysts

The frequency of additional abnormalities in chromosomally normal and trisomy 18 fetuses with CPCs is shown in Table 2.16 (Snijders *et al* 1994).

Table 2.16 Frequency of additional abnormalities in 332 fetuses with choroid plexus cysts and an apparently normal karyotype and in 38 fetuses with trisomy 18 and choroid plexus cysts at 16–23 weeks of gestation (Snijders *et al* 1994b).

Abnormality	Normal karyotype			Trisomy 18		
	Total	Abnormalities 1	2	Total	Abnormalities 1	≥2
	n=332	n=46	n=15	n=38	n=2	n=35
Clenched hand	1 (0.3%)	-	1	24 (63%)	-	24
Strawberry-shaped head	1 (0.3%)	-	1	24 (63%)	-	24
Heart defect	1 (0.3%)	-	1	17 (45%)	-	17
Micrognathia	1 (0.3%)	-	1	15 (39%)	-	15
Exomphalos	1 (0.3%)	-	1	11 (29%)	-	10
Talipes equinovarus	3 (0.9%)	1	2	8 (21%)	-	8
Facial cleft	-	-	-	5 (13%)	-	5
Rocker-bottom feet	-	-	-	5 (13%)	-	5
Nuchal oedema	4 (1.2%)	2	2	4 (11%)	-	4
Multicystic kidneys	3 (0.9%)	1	2	4 (11%)	-	4
Severe hydronephrosis	2 (0.6%)	1	1	0 (0%)	-	-
Absent stomach bubble	-	-	-	4 (11%)	-	4
Diaphragmatic hernia	-	-	-	3 (8%)	-	3
Hydrops fetalis	-	-	-	2 (3%)	-	2
Posterior fossa cyst	-	-	-	2 (3%)	-	2
Absent corpus callosum	-	-	-	1 (2%)	-	1
Cystic adenomatoid malf.	-	-	-	1 (2%)	-	1
Spina bifida	-	-	-	1 (2%)	-	1
Kyphoscoliosis	2 (0.6%)	1	1	0 (0%)	-	-
Small for gestational age	8 (2.4%)	4	4	17 (45%)	-	17
Brachycephaly	8 (2.4%)	5	3	13 (34%)	2	11
Short femur	7 (2.1%)	3	4	9 (24%)	-	9
Pylectasia	26 (7.8%)	21	5	10 (26%)	-	10
Ventriculomegaly	9 (2.7%)	7	2	5 (13%)	-	5
Microcephaly	2 (0.6%)	-	2	2 (5%)	-	2

Chromosomally normal fetuses

In a group of 332 chromosomally normal fetuses with CPCs, Snijders *et al* (1994) reported that the frequency of additional abnormalities was 18%. Although this is much higher than the

5% from other reports (Table 2.14), in these studies no details were provided as to which abnormalities were systematically searched for. If biometrical abnormalities were considered, the frequency should have been higher; by definition, for each parameter, 5% of the normal population will have values outside the 95% confidence interval of the normal range. In the study of Snijders *et al* (1994b), if biometrical abnormalities were excluded, the frequency of additional defects was 4% (Table 2.16).

Trisomy 18 fetuses

In the 38 trisomy 18 fetuses with CPCs, the frequency of additional abnormalities was 97% (Table 2.16), whereas in the combined group of 22 fetuses from the screening studies (see Table 2.14), only 14 (64%) had additional abnormalities.

The most likely explanation for this difference is that in the Harris Birthright Research Centre for Fetal Medicine there has been a high awareness for many years of the possible association between CPCs and trisomy 18 (Nicolaides *et al* 1986), and therefore, whenever CPCs were observed, a systematic search for additional abnormalities was undertaken.

Therefore, in the 38 trisomy 18 fetuses with CPCs, 2.6% had no other abnormalities, 5.3% had one additional abnormality and 92.1% had at least two additional abnormalities (Table 2.17). The corresponding percentages for the 332 chromosomally normal fetuses with CPCs were 81.6%, 13.9% and 4.5% (Table 2.17).

Table 2.17 Number of additional abnormalities in 370 fetuses with choroid plexus cysts in trisomy 18 fetuses or in chromosomally normal fetuses. The likelihood ratio is the ratio of frequency with which 0, 1 or ≥2 additional abnormalities were observed in the group with trisomy 18 to the respective frequencies in the chromosomally normal group.

Additional abnormalities	Trisomy 18 (n=38)	Normal (n=332)	Likelihood ratio
0	1 (2.6%)	271 (81.6%)	0.032
1	2 (5.3%)	46 (13.9%)	0.379
≥2	35 (92.1%)	15 (4.5%)	20.39

On the basis of these data it can be calculated that, in fetuses with CPCs, the likelihood ratio of trisomy 18 is 0.03 if the CPCs are isolated, 0.4 if there is one additional abnormality and 20.5 if there are two or more additional abnormalities.

Calculation of risks

In the calculation of risks for trisomy 18 in mid-trimester fetuses with CPCs the following assumptions were made: (i) the risk for trisomy 18 increases with advancing maternal age, (ii) the prevalence of CPCs in the general population is approximately 1%, and (iii) at mid-gestation the incidence of CPCs in fetuses with trisomy 18 is approximately 50%, (iv) within the group of fetuses with CPCs, the likelihood ratio for trisomy 18 increases with the number of additional abnormalities.

The estimated maternal age-related risks for trisomy 18 in the presence of fetal CPCs and additional abnormalities are shown in Table 2.13.

To illustrate how the calculations were made, the example of a 32 year old woman was used. The maternal age-related risk for trisomy 18 at 20 weeks of gestation is 1/2,114. Since CPCs are present in 50% of fetuses with trisomy 18, if no CPCs are found the risk is 0.5/2,114 or 1/4,228. Since 1% of all fetuses have CPCs and 50% of fetuses with trisomy 18 have CPCs, the incidence of trisomy 18 in the presence of fetal CPCs is 0.50/(2,114 x 0.01) or 1/42.

To derive risks for fetuses with and without additional abnormalities, overall risks for fetuses with CPCs were expressed as odds ratios (number of abnormal pregnancies to number of normal pregnancies) and the left hand side of the odds ratio was multiplied by the appropriate likelihood ratio (Table 2.18).

Recommendation

The detection of fetal CPCs should stimulate the sonographer to search for the other features of trisomy 18: strawberry-shaped head, ventriculomegaly, absent corpus callosum, enlarged cisterna magna, facial cleft, micrognathia, nuchal oedema, cardiac defect, diaphragmatic hernia, oesophageal atresia, renal defects, exomphalos, short limbs, talipes or rocker-bottom feet, overlapping fingers, growth retardation.

If the cysts are apparently isolated, the risk for trisomy 18 is only marginally increased and maternal age should be the main factor in deciding whether or not fetal karyotyping should be performed.

If one additional abnormality is found, the maternal age-related risk is increased by about 20 times, so that even for a 22 year old the risk for trisomy 18 (1/249) is similar to the risk for trisomy 21 in a 35 year old (1/274); in this respect, it may be considered rational to offer such patients the option of karyotyping.

If two or more additional abnormalities are found, the risk is increased by almost 1,000 times and karyotyping should be offered irrespective of maternal age.

Table 2.18 Estimates of the risk for trisomy 18 (1/number in the table) in 20–24 week fetuses with isolated choroid plexus cysts (CPCs) and in those with one and two or more, additional abnormalities.

Maternal age (yrs)	Total population	Choroid plexus cysts		Additional abnormalities		
		absent	present	0	1	>2
20	6472	12944	129	4015	341	6
22	6233	12466	125	3950	328	6
24	5848	11696	117	3628	308	6
26	5267	10534	105	3267	277	5
28	4475	8950	90	2776	236	4
30	3529	7058	71	2189	186	3
32	2563	5126	51	1590	135	3
34	1722	3444	34	1068	91	2
36	1086	2172	22	674	57	<2
38	655	1310	13	406	34	<2
40	384	768	8	238	20	<2
42	221	442	4	137	12	<2
44	125	250	3	78	7	<2
46	71	142	1	44	4	<2

THE EXAMPLE OF MILD HYDRONEPHROSIS AND TRISOMY 21

Pyelectasia, or mild hydronephrosis, is found in a wide variety of chromosomal defects, unlike choroid plexus cysts which are mainly associated with trisomy 18. In the combined data from five studies on a total of 631 fetuses with mild hydronephrosis, the prevalence of chromosomal defects was 8% (Table 2.19).

Table 2.19 Studies examining the prevalence of chromosomal defects in fetuses with mild hydronephrosis according to the presence or absence of additional abnormalities.

Author		Incidence of chromosomal defects						
	N	Total	Isolated	Multiple	21	18	13	Oth
Benacerraf et al (90b)	210	7 (3%)	?	?	7			
Van Zalen-Sprock et al (91)	21	1 (5%)	1/21	-	1			
Nicolaides et al (92b)	258	35 (4%)	5/163	30/95	15	6	8	6
Corteville et al (92)	127	7 (6%)	0/116	7/11	4			3
Wilson et al (92)	15	0 (0%)	0/10	0/5				
Total	631	50 (8%)	2%	33%	27	6	8	9

Although the majority of fetuses with chromosomal defects had additional abnormalities, even in those fetuses with apparently isolated hydronephrosis the prevalence of chromosomal defects was 2%. However, it is uncertain whether this high frequency truly reflects an increased risk over that expected on the basis of the maternal age and gestational age distributions of the populations examined.

This section demonstrates an approach for evaluating the possible significance of chromosomal 'markers' such as mild hydro-nephrosis and the data are derived from 1177 fetuses that were examined at the Harris Birthright Research Centre for Fetal Medicine during an 8-year period (1986–1994) (Snijders et al 1995b).

The diagnosis of mild hydronephrosis was based on the demonstration of a minimum antero-posterior pelvic diameter of 4 mm with no calyceal dilatation and normal renal cortical echogenicity and bladder. The median gestation was 20 weeks (range 16–26), and the median maternal age was 30 years (range 15–44 years).

Total frequency of chromosomal defects

The fetal karyotype was abnormal in 7.3% of the cases and the most common chromosomal defects were trisomies 21, 18 and 13 (Table 2.20). However, this high prevalence of chromosomal defects is a mere consequence of the preselection of patients referred to a specialist centre, rather than the true significance of mild hydronephrosis.

Table 2.20 Chromosomal defects in 1,177 fetuses with mild hydronephrosis at the Harris Birthright Research Centre for Fetal Medicine.

Chromosomal defect	N	%
Trisomies		
21	37	3.14
18	13	1.10
13	18	1.53
20	1	0.08
8 mosaic	1	0.08
5p	1	0.08
12p	1	0.08
Unbalanced translocations		
13;14	1	0.08
13;21	1	0.08
7;8	1	0.08
Deletions		
13q	1	0.08
14q	2	0.17
Turner syndrome	6	0.51
Triploidy	2	0.17
Total	**86**	**7.31**

Frequency of chromosomal defects and number of abnormalities

In the 1,177 fetuses with mild hydronephrosis, the prevalence of chromosomal defects increased with the number of additional abnormalities. In the 805 cases with apparently isolated hydronephrosis, the prevalence was 1.1%, whereas in those with one, two and three or more additional defects the prevalences were 5.4%, 22.9% and 63.3%, respectively (Figure 2.11).

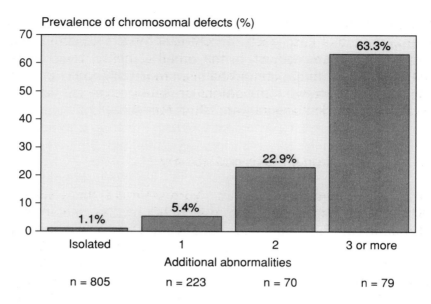

Figure 2.11 Prevalence of chromosomal defects in fetuses with mild hydronephrosis according to the number of additional abnormalities

Pattern of abnormalities

For each chromosomal defect, there was a characteristic pattern of associated abnormalities (see Chapter 1). For example, both fetuses with triploidy had severe asymmetrical intrauterine growth retardation and five of the six fetuses with Turner syndrome had cystic hygromata. All 13 fetuses with trisomy 18, in addition to the mild hydronephrosis, had at least three other abnormalities, such as choroid plexus or posterior fossa cysts, nuchal oedema, facial cleft, micrognathia, cardiac abnormalities, diaphragmatic hernia, oesophageal atresia, exomphalos, short limbs, talipes or overlapping fingers. Similarly, in trisomy 13, the most common associated abnormalities were holoprosencephaly, facial cleft, nuchal oedema, cardiac and digital; however, unlike trisomy 18, where all fetuses had at least three additional abnormalities, in trisomy 13, two fetuses had only one additional abnormality, one case with nuchal oedema and another with a cardiac abnormality.

In five of the 37 fetuses with trisomy 21, the only abnormal finding was mild hydronephrosis. In another 10 cases, there was only one additional abnormality; four with clinodactyly, three with nuchal oedema, and one case each of ventriculomegaly, choroid plexus cysts and echogenic bowel. In the other 22 cases, there were at least two additional abnormalities, most commonly nuchal oedema, clinodactyly, atrioventricular septal defects, echogenic bowel, mild ventriculomegaly and short femur.

Isolated mild hydronephrosis and trisomy 21

In the 805 fetuses with isolated hydronephrosis there were five (0.62%) with trisomy 21. On the basis of the maternal age distribution of this population and estimates of maternal and gestational age-specific risks for trisomy 21 (see Table 2.2), the expected number of fetuses with trisomy 21 was three (0.40%). The difference between the observed and expected frequency of trisomy 21 in this group of 805 fetuses was not significant. To demonstrate that such a difference is significant (power 80%), it would be necessary to investigate a minimum of 24,741 fetuses with mild hydronephrosis. Since the prevalence of mild hydronephrosis at 20 weeks of gestation is about 2% (Corteville *et al* 1992), in order to complete such a study it would be necessary to scan at least one million pregnancies. In the meantime, there are two options in counselling parents. First, they could be told that the presence of mild hydronephrosis does not increase significantly the risk that the fetus has trisomy 21. Alternatively, the risk is 1.6 times higher than the maternal age and gestational age-related risk. This factor of 1.6 is derived by dividing the observed (0.62%) by the expected (0.40%) frequency in the 805 fetuses in the above study (Table 2.21).

Table 2.21 Frequency of trisomy 21 in 1177 fetuses with mild hydronephrosis in relation to the presence of additional abnormalities. The expected frequency in each subgroup was derived from the maternal age and gestational age distribution of the populations and the age-specific risk for trisomy 21.

Additional abnormalities		Observed frequency N	%	Expected frequency N	%	Observed / expected
0	(n=805)	5	0.62	3.20	0.40	1.6
1	(n=223)	10	4.48	0.67	0.30	14.9
2	(n=70)	10	14.29	0.22	0.31	46.1
≥ 3	(n=79)	12	15.19	0.21	0.27	56.3

Similarly, the observed to expected ratios for trisomy 21 in fetuses with mild hydronephrosis and one, two and three or more additional abnormalities are 14.9, 46.1 and 56.3, respectively (Table 2.21).

To derive risks for trisomy 21 in 20 week gestation fetuses with mild hydronephrosis in the absence and presence of additional abnormalities, the maternal age-related risks at this gestation (see Table 2.2) are multiplied by the appropriate observed to expected ratio (Table 2.21). The results are illustrated in Figure 2.12.

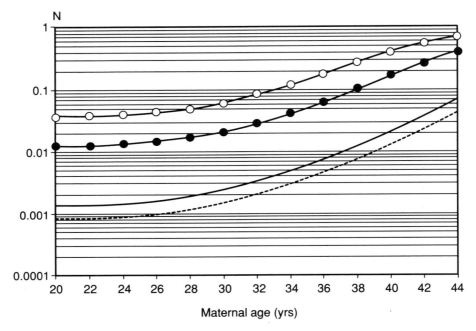

Figure 2.12 Maternal age-related risk for trisomy 21 at 20 weeks of gestation (- - -) and the risks in the presence of isolated mild hydronephrosis (——), and with one (●), two or more (○) additional abnormalities.

Recommendation

The detection of fetal mild hydronephrosis should stimulate the sonographer to search for the other abnormalities. It should be remembered that, if there is an underlying chromosomal defect, such as trisomy 18, this may be associated with multiple easily detectable abnormalities, but if the defect is trisomy 21, the other abnormalities are usually subtle.

For apparently isolated mild hydronephrosis, there may be a small increase in maternal age and gestational age-related risk for trisomy 21. If the arbitrary level of risk for offering invasive testing is taken to be that based on a maternal age of 37 years, this risk at 20 weeks of gestation is 1/168 (see Table 2.2). In the presence of apparently isolated mild hydronephrosis, the risk of 1/168 is reached only if the maternal age is at least 35 years.

When there is one additional abnormality, the risk even for a 20 year old woman increases from 1/1175 to 1/80; with two additional abnormalities the risk is increased to 1/26, and with three or more additional abnormalities the risk is 1/22.

THE EXAMPLE OF EXOMPHALOS AND TRISOMIES 18 AND 13

Ultrasound studies examining the association between fetal abnormalities and chromosomal defects often fail to take into account the maternal age and gestational age distribution of their population and inevitably report conflicting results. For example, the reported prevalence of chromosomal defects in mid-trimester fetuses with exomphalos varies from 10% to 66% (see Table 1.15).

Exomphalos, found in about one per 3000 births, is a correctable malformation and, when the condition is isolated, the survival rate is more than 90%. However, a high proportion of fetuses with exomphalos have chromosomal defects, most commonly trisomies 18 or 13 (see Table 1.15).

The frequency of these chromosomal defects increases with maternal age and decreases with gestation, because they are associated with a high rate of intrauterine lethality (see Tables 2.3 and 2.4). Consequently, both the prevalence of exomphalos and the prevalence of associated trisomies would be expected to increase with maternal age and decrease with advancing gestation. This section demonstrates the necessary methodology to test this hypothesis.

First trimester screening study

In an ultrasound screening study at 11–14 weeks of gestation involving 15,726 viable, singleton pregnancies, the prevalence of exomphalos was 0.11% (18 cases). A minimum crown–rump length of 43 mm was selected to exclude cases of physiological herniation of bowel into the umbilical cord. In the 18 cases of exomphalos there were nine with trisomy 18, one with trisomy 13 and one with triploidy (Snijders *et al* 1995c).

In the screened population, the total observed numbers of trisomy 18, trisomy 13 and triploidy were 40, 11 and 8, respectively. These numbers were similar to the numbers expected on the basis of the maternal and gestational age distribution of this population (33, 10 and 8, respectively).

To calculate the expected number of cases with chromosomal defects, the maternal age distribution and estimates of maternal and gestational age-specific risks were used (see Tables 2.3 and 2.4, Figure 2.10). For each year of maternal age, the gestation-specific incidence of trisomy 18, trisomy 13, and triploidy were multiplied with the number of women in that age group. The sum of numbers for each year of maternal age and each gestation provided the expected total. The prevalence of exomphalos in fetuses with trisomy 18 was 22.5%, in fetuses with trisomy 13 it was 9.1% and in those with triploidy it was 12.5%, whereas in those with no evidence of these chromosomal defects the incidence was 0.045% (Table 2.22).

Table 2.22 Observed prevalences of trisomy 18, trisomy 13, triploidy and exomphalos in an ultrasound screening study at 11–14 weeks of gestation involving 15,726 women with a median age of 33 years. In the last column is the percentage of fetuses with exomphalos in each karyotype group.

Karyotype	Total	Exomphalos	
		N	%
Trisomy 18	40	9	22.500
Trisomy 13	11	1	9.091
Triploidy	8	1	12.500
Other	15,667	7	0.045
Total	**15,726**	**18**	**0.114**

Expected frequencies in an unselected population

The median maternal age of the screened population was 33 years, which was higher than the median age of all deliveries in England and Wales or the United States of America (Figure 2.13). To calculate the expected number of cases with trisomy 18, trisomy 13, and triploidy of all deliveries in England and Wales, the maternal age distribution (OPCS) and estimates of maternal and gestational age-specific risks were used (Table 2.23).

Table 2.23 Estimates for the number of fetuses with trisomy 18 or trisomy 13 at different stages of pregnancy in an unselected population of 100,000 pregnancies. The total number of cases in each age bracket (N) was derived from the distribution of maternal age for all deliveries in England and Wales in 1992 (OPCS).

Maternal age (yrs)	N	Trisomy 18			Trisomy 13		
		12 wk	20 wk	Birth	12 wk	20 wk	Birth
<25	30,800	12.1	4.9	2.7	3.9	1.8	0.8
25-29	35,534	18.3	7.5	3.2	5.9	2.8	1.2
30-34	24,102	23.0	9.3	4.1	7.4	3.5	1.5
35-39	8,132	22.1	8.9	3.9	7.1	3.4	1.5
40-44	1,373	12.7	5.2	2.2	4.1	1.9	0.8
≥45	59	1.8	0.7	0.3	0.6	0.3	0.1
Total	**100,000**	**90.0**	**36.5**	**16.4**	**29.0**	**13.7**	**5.9**

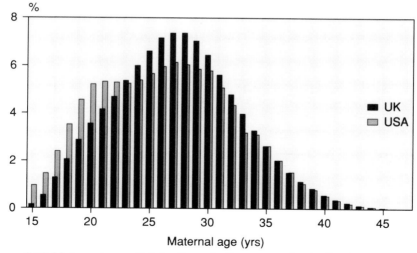

Figure 2.13 Maternal age distribution of all pregnancies in England and Wales (OPCS 1993) and the United States of America (Department of Health 1993).

Table 2.24 Expected frequencies of trisomy 18, trisomy 13 and triploidy in unselected populations at 12 and 20 weeks of gestation and in live births. The total numbers in the groups with a chromosomal defect were multiplied by the observed prevalences of exomphalos (Exom) in the screening study at 11–14 weeks of gestation. In the group without evidence of trisomy 18, trisomy 13 or triploidy the prevalence of exomphalos at 12 weeks was assumed to be 0.045% and at 20 weeks and in live births it was assumed to be 0.025%. The latter prevalence was derived on the basis of the assumption that the fetuses with lethal additional abnormalities will have died before 20 weeks of gestation.

Karyotype	12 weeks		20 weeks		Live births	
	N	Exom	N	Exom	N	Exom
Trisomy 18	90	20.3	36.5	8.1	16.4	3.7
Trisomy 13	29	2.6	13.7	1.2	5.9	0.5
Triploidy	50	6.3	1.4	0.2	0.0	0.0
Other	99,831	45.0	99,949	25.0	99,978	25.0
Total	**100,000**	**74.2**	**100,000**	**34.5**	**100,000**	**29.2**

To derive an estimate for the number of cases with exomphalos in each karyotype group (Table 2.24), the expected number of cases (Table 2.23) was multiplied by the prevalence of exomphalos observed in the screening study at 11–14 weeks of gestation (Table 2.22).

Therefore, in an unselected population of 100,000 deliveries with the maternal age distribution of England and Wales, which is very similar to that in the United States of America, the expected number of fetuses with exomphalos at 12 weeks of gestation is 74 (Table 2.23).

Second trimester study on referred patients

During a 6-year period, a total of 153 pregnancies with fetal exomphalos diagnosed by routine ultrasound examination at 16–26 weeks of gestation were referred for fetal karyotyping to the Harris Birthright Research Centre for Fetal Medicine.

The median maternal age was 29 (16–48) years and the fetal karyotype was abnormal in 49 cases, including 34 (22.2%) with trisomy 18, eight (5.2%) with trisomy 13 and one (0.7%) with triploidy (Table 2.22).

These observed frequencies of trisomies and triploidy in the referred population are similar to those derived for an unselected population.

Thus, as shown in Table 2.21, in an unselected population of 100,000 pregnancies at 20 weeks of gestation, the total expected number of fetuses with exomphalos is about 35; the estimated incidence of trisomy 18, trisomy 13 and triploidy in these 35 fetuses is 23.4%, 3.5% and 0.6%, respectively (Table 2.25).

Table 2.25 Observed frequencies of trisomy 18, trisomy 13 and triploidy in 153 fetuses with exomphalos at 16–26 weeks of gestation and expected frequencies on the basis of (i) the age distribution of all deliveries in England and Wales in 1992, (ii) estimates for maternal and gestational age-specific risks for chromosomal defects and (iii) prevalences of exomphalos in the first trimester of pregnancy.

Karyotype	Observed	Expected
Trisomy 18	22.2%	23.4%
Trisomy 13	5.2%	3.5%
Triploidy	0.7%	0.6%
Total	**28.1%**	**27.5%**

These data, that the prevalence of chromosomal defects in fetuses with exomphalos investigated in a tertiary referral centre is similar to that expected on the basis of the maternal age and gestational age distribution of the patients, suggest that the patients with exomphalos examined in a referral centre are representative of an unselected population of fetuses with this abnormality.

These findings are likely to be the consequence of (i) easy diagnosis of all or most cases of exomphalos at routine ultrasound examination, and (ii) that all or most cases of exomphalos are referred for fetal karyotyping.

For example, if only fetuses with the most severe types of exomphalos were diagnosed, then the observed incidence of chromosomal defects would have been lower than the expected because the incidence of chromosomal defects is higher in those cases where the exomphalos sac contains only bowel rather than liver and other organs. Similarly, if in the routine centres there was patient preselection, so that fetuses with multiple additional abnormalities were more likely to be referred for fetal karyotyping rather than those with isolated exomphalos, then the observed incidence of chromosomal defects in reports from referral centres would have been higher than expected.

Reported incidence in postnatal studies

In six studies on neonates with exomphalos, trisomy 18 or 13 was diagnosed in 9.3% of cases (Table 2.26), which was significantly lower than the 14.4% expected for an unselected population (Table 2.27). Thus, as shown in Table 2.24, in an unselected population of 100,000 live births, the total expected number of babies with exomphalos is about 29; the estimated frequencies of trisomies 18 and 13 in these 29 fetuses are 12.7% and 1.7%, respectively.

Table 2.26 Studies reporting the frequency of chromosomal defects in neonates with exomphalos.

Author	N	Trisomy 18	Trisomy 13
Carpenter *et al* 84	25	0 (0%)	1 (4%)
Kirk & Wah 83	38	2 (5%)	1 (3%)
Wladimiroff *et al* 83	46	?3 (7%)	?2 (4%)
Mabogunje *et al* 84	57	3 (5%)	2 (4%)
Hasan & Hermansen 86	17	1 (6%)	1 (6%)
Calzolari *et al* 93	116	6 (5%)	6 (5%)
Total	**299**	**15 (5.0%)**	**13 (4.3%)**

Table 2.27 Observed frequencies of trisomy 18, trisomy 13 and triploidy in 299 neonates with exomphalos and expected frequencies on the basis of (i) the age distribution of all deliveries in England and Wales in 1992, (ii) estimates for maternal and gestational age-specific risks for chromosomal defects and (iii) prevalences of exomphalos in the first trimester of pregnancy.

Karyotype	Observed	Expected
Trisomy 18	5.0%	12.7%
Trisomy 13	4.3%	1.7%
Triploidy	0.0%	0.0%
Total	**9.3%**	**14.4%**

The most likely explanation for the finding, that the frequency of chromosomal defects in neonates with exomphalos is lower than expected on the basis of the maternal age and gestational age distribution of an unselected population, is that the published series are mainly from neonatal surgical units. Babies with obvious features of lethal chromosomal abnormalities born at non-specialist centres are unlikely to be referred for neonatal surgery.

THE EXAMPLE OF FACIAL CLEFT AND TRISOMIES 18 AND 13

In contrast to exomphalos, which is easy to diagnose at routine ultrasound examination, prenatal diagnosis of facial cleft is difficult and the majority of cases are missed. Thus, in two screening studies involving a total of 24,802 patients, the prevalence of facial cleft was 0.125% and routine ultrasound examination identified only 23% of the fetuses (Table 2.28).

Table 2.28 Studies providing data on the prevalence of facial cleft in the second trimester of pregnancy.

Study	N	Facial cleft	
		Prevalence	% detected
Levi *et al* 91	16,370	0.147%	5/24 (21%)
Chitty *et al* 91	8,432	0.083%	2/7 (29%)
Total	**24,802**	**0.125%**	**7/31 (23%)**

Since fetuses with additional multiple abnormalities are more likely to be identified than those with an isolated facial cleft, it is expected that antenatal studies would overestimate the frequency of associated chromosomal defects.

Furthermore, with improving quality of ultrasound equipment and standards of scanning, it is likely that more cases of isolated facial cleft would be identified and consequently, the observed frequency of chromosomal defects would decrease with time.

This section demonstrates the necessary methodology to test this hypothesis.

Second trimester study on referred patients

Prevalence of chromosomal defects in fetuses with a facial cleft

During a 7-year period a total of 111 pregnancies with fetal facial cleft diagnosed by routine ultrasound examination at 16–26 weeks of gestation were referred for fetal karyotyping to the Harris Birthright Research Centre for Fetal Medicine (Snijders *et al* 1995d).

In 41 (37%) of the cases the facial cleft was isolated and in 70 (63%) there were multiple additional abnormalities. In 39 of the latter group (35% of the total), there was an associated chromosomal defect; trisomy 18 (n=7), trisomy 13 (n=22), unbalanced translocation between chromosomes 13 and 14 (n=3) and one case each of trisomy 21, trisomy 22, partial trisomy 4q, deletion 21q, deletion 4p, inversion of chromosome 9 and triploidy.

During the first 4-year period of the study, in 25% of the fetuses with facial clefts there were no other detectable abnormalities and the overall prevalence of chromosomal defects was 42% (Table 2.29). In the subsequent 3 years, the proportion of fetuses with an isolated facial cleft doubled and the overall prevalence of associated chromosomal defects decreased.

Table 2.29 Findings in fetuses with a facial cleft that were referred to the Harris Birthright Research Centre for Fetal Medicine between 1988 and 1994.

Period	N	Isolated	Abnormal karyotype
1988-1991	57	14 (25%)	24 (42%)
1992-1994	54	27 (50%)	15 (28%)
Total	**111**	**41 (37%)**	**39 (35%)**

Prevalence of facial cleft in trisomic fetuses

During the same 7-year period (1988–1994), in the Harris Birthright Research Centre for Fetal Medicine, trisomy 18 was diagnosed in 102 fetuses and trisomy 13 in 54. The prevalence of facial cleft in fetuses with trisomy 18 at 16–26 weeks of gestation was 6.9% (7 of 102) and in those with trisomy 13 it was 40.7% (22 of 54).

Expected prevalence in an unselected population

The distribution of maternal age for all deliveries in England and Wales (see Figure 2.11) and estimates for the prevalences of trisomies 18 and 13 at 20 weeks of gestation (see Tables 2.3 and 2.4) were used to calculate the total number of fetuses with trisomies 18 and 13 per 100,000 pregnancies (Table 2.30).

Table 2.30 Estimates for the total number of fetuses with a facial cleft, the total number of fetuses with trisomy 18, the number of fetuses with trisomy 18 and a facial cleft, the total number of fetuses with trisomy 13 and the number with trisomy 13 and facial cleft at 20 weeks of gestation in an unselected population of 100,000 pregnancies. The total number of cases in each age bracket (N) was derived from the distribution of maternal age for all deliveries in England and Wales in 1992 (OPCS) and the overall frequency of facial cleft was assumed to be 0.125% (see Table 2.25). The total numbers of trisomies 18 and 13 were derived from the age-related risks for these trisomies at 20 weeks of gestation (see Tables 2.3 and 2.4) and the assumption that in fetuses with trisomies 18 and 13 the prevalence of facial cleft is 6.9% and 40.7%, respectively.

Maternal age (yrs)	All pregnancies		Trisomy 18		Trisomy 13	
	Total	Cleft	Total	Cleft	Total	Cleft
<25	30,800	38.5	4.9	0.34	1.8	0.73
25-29	35,534	44.4	7.5	0.52	2.8	1.14
30-34	24,102	30.2	9.3	0.64	3.5	1.42
35-39	8,132	10.2	8.9	0.61	3.4	1.38
40-44	1,373	1.7	5.2	0.36	1.9	0.77
≥45	59	0.07	0.7	0.05	0.3	0.12
Total	**100,000**	**125.0**	**36.5**	**2.52**	**13.7**	**5.56**

On the assumption that facial cleft is present in 0.125% of all fetuses (see Table 2.28), in 6.9% of those with trisomy 18 and in 40.7% of those with trisomy 13 (see section above), then in an unselected population where all cases of fetal facial cleft are detected, the prevalence of trisomies 18 and 13 is 6.5% (Table 2.30).

The findings, that the prevalence of chromosomal defects in fetuses with facial cleft investigated in a tertiary referral centre (35%) is much higher than that expected in all fetuses with facial cleft in an unselected population (6.5%), demonstrate that the patients with facial cleft examined in a referral centre are preselected.

These findings are compatible with the results of the screening studies that the majority of fetuses with facial cleft are not presently detectable at routine ultrasound examination. Furthermore, the results suggest that those that are diagnosed are pre-selected by the presence of additional multi-system abnormalities.

CALCULATION OF RISKS FOR TRISOMY 21 BY COMBINING DATA ON SEVERAL SONOGRAPHIC MARKERS

Several second trimester ultrasonographic markers have been investigated for their value in identifying fetuses with trisomy 21. Examples of those that have been studied in detail are nuchal fold thickness or nuchal oedema, mild hydronephrosis or pylectasia, relative shortening of the femur and, more recently, hyperechogenic bowel.

This section illustrates how data reported in the literature could be used to derive estimates of risks and it points out which questions need to be answered before clinically useful estimates become available.

In the calculation of adjusted risk, the likelihood ratio is first derived by dividing the prevalence of a given marker in trisomy 21 by the prevalence in normal fetuses. The likelihood ratio is then multiplied by the background risk which is expressed as an odds ratio.

Nuchal fold thickening

The combined data from seven large studies indicate that the prevalence of nuchal fold thickness ≥6 mm in trisomy 21 fetuses is 35%, compared to 0.73% in normal fetuses (Table 2.31). Therefore, the likelihood ratio for this sonographic marker is 48.

Five of the seven studies reported on the presence of additional abnormalities in the trisomic fetuses, and from these studies 14% of trisomy 21 fetuses had increased nuchal thickness as the only sonographic finding. Consequently, the likelihood ratio for trisomy 21 in the presence of apparently isolated increased nuchal thickness is 14/0.73 or 19.

Table 2.31 Prevalence of nuchal fold thickness ≥6 mm in trisomy 21 and normal fetuses. The frequency of apparently isolated increase in nuchal fold thickness in trisomy 21 fetuses was provided in only five of the studies [ ].

	Trisomy 21	Normal	Likelihood ratio
Nyberg *et al* 90	4/25 (16%) ?	10/3500 (0.29%)	55
DeVore & Alfi 93	7/35 (20%) [0]	14/2772 (0.51%)	39
Benacerraf *et al* 87	9/21 (43%) [0]	4/3804 (0.10%)	430
Kirk *et al* 92	9/19 (47%) [6]	18/7093 (0.30%)	157
Watson *et al* 94	7/14 (50%) [4]	27/1381 (1.96%)	25
Crane & Gray 91	12/16 (75%) [5]	35/3322 (1.05%)	71
Grandjean *et al* 95	11/39 (29%) ?	70/2381 (2.94%)	10
Total	**59/169 (35%)**	**178/24,253 (0.73%)**	**48**
Isolated	**15/105 (14%)**		**19**

Hyperechogenic bowel

The combined data from four studies indicate that the prevalence of hyperechogenic bowel in fetuses with trisomy 21 is 11%, compared to 0.5% in normal fetuses (Table 2.32). Therefore, the likelihood ratio for this sonographic marker is 22.

In 15 of the 20 fetuses with trisomy 21 and hyperechogenic bowel, there were additional abnormalities. Consequently, the likelihood ratio for trisomy 21 of apparently isolated hyperechogenic bowel is 2.7/0.49 or 5.5.

Table 2.32 Prevalence of hyperechogenic bowel in trisomy 21 and normal fetuses. Apparently isolated hyperechogenic bowel [ ] was found in 2.7% of trisomy 21 fetuses.

	Trisomy 21	Normal	Likelihood ratio
Dicke & Crane 92	0/47 (0.0) [0]	30/12,776 (0.23)	?
Nyberg *et al* 93b	8/68 (11.8) [3]	55/6781 (0.81)	14.6
Bromley *et al* 94	6/48 (12.5) [0]	50/8680 (0.58)	21.6
Scioscia *et al* 92	6/19 (31.6) [2]	16/2300 (0.70)	45.1
Total	**20/182 (11.0)**	**151/30,537 (0.49)**	**22.4**
Isolated	**5/182 (2.7)**		**5.5**

Relative shortening of the femur

Relative shortening of the femur has been defined either as a measurement of femur below the 5th centile, as a ratio of biparietal diameter to femur length above the 95th centile, or as a ratio of the observed to expected femur length for gestation above 0.91. The combined data from eight studies indicate that the prevalence of relatively short femur in fetuses with trisomy 21 is 28%, compared to 4.3% in normal fetuses (Table 2.33). Therefore, the likelihood ratio for this sonographic marker is 6.5. Seven of the studies did not provide data on the presence or absence of additional abnormalities. Benacerraf *et al* (1987) reported that 42% of fetuses with trisomy 21 and relative shortening of the femur had no apparent additional abnormalities. On the basis of these data, it was derived that the prevalence of isolated relative shortening of the femur in fetuses with trisomy 21 is 10% (0.042 × 66/267) which would give a likelihood ratio of 10/4.3 or 2.3.

Table 2.33 Prevalence relative shortening of the femur in trisomy 21 and normal fetuses. It was estimated that relatively short femur may be an apparently isolated finding in 10% of fetuses with trisomy 21.

	Trisomy 21	Normal	Likelihood ratio
Lockwood *et al* 87	6/42 (14%)	163/4949 (3.3)	4.2
Dicke *et al* 89	6/33 (18%)	7/177 (4.0)	4.5
Rodis *et al* 91	2/11 (18%)	95/1890 (5.0)	3.6
Cuckle *et al* 89	20/83 (24%)	84/1340 (6.3)	3.8
Nyberg *et al* 93c	11/45 (24%)	44/942 (4.7)	5.1
Hill *et al* 89	8/22 (36%)	20/286 (7.0)	5.1
Ginsberg *et al* 90	5/11 (45%)	14/212 (6.6)	6.8
Benacerraf *et al* 87	19/28 (68%)	4/192 (2.0)	34.0
Total	**77/275 (28%)**	**431/9988 (4.3)**	**6.5**
Isolated	**~10%**		**2.3**

Mild hydronephrosis or pylectasia

The combined data from two studies indicate that the prevalence of mild hydronephrosis in trisomy 21 fetuses is 21%, compared to 2.5% in normal fetuses (Table 2.34). Therefore, the likelihood ratio for this sonographic marker is 8.4. The study of Corteville *et al* (1992) provided data on the presence of additional abnormalities, which were present in three of the four trisomic fetuses with mild hydronephrosis. Therefore, the likelihood ratio for trisomy 21 in the presence of apparently isolated mild hydronephrosis is 4/2.5 or 1.5. This ratio is almost identical to the value of 1.6 derived in our study (see the example of mild hydronephrosis).

Table 2.34 Prevalence of mild hydronephrosis in trisomy 21 and normal fetuses. The frequency of apparently isolated hydronephrosis in trisomy 21 fetuses was provided in one of the studies [ ].

	Trisomy 21	Normal	Likelihood ratio
Benacerraf *et al* 90	7/29 (24)	210/7400 (2.8)	8.6
Corteville *et al* 92	4/23 (17) [1]	120/5876 (2.0)	8.7
Total	11/52 (21)	330/13,276 (2.5)	8.4
Isolated	1/23 (4)		1.5

Provisional estimates of risks in the presence of markers

Table 2.35 provides the maternal age-related risk for trisomy 21 at 20 weeks of gestation and the estimated adjusted risks in the presence of apparently isolated markers. When two or more of these markers are present, a new likelihood ratio is derived by multiplying the ratios for the individual markers. For example, in the presence of both mild hydronephrosis and relatively short femur, the likelihood ratio is 1.5 × 2.3 or 3.45 and therefore the risk for a 30-year-old woman at 20 weeks of gestation is increased from 1:689 (or 1/690) to 3.45:689 or 1:200 (or 1/201).

Provisional estimates of risks in the absence of markers

On the basis of the data provided in Tables 2.31-2.34, apparently isolated nuchal fold thickness ≥6 mm, hyperechogenic bowel, relatively short femur or mild hydronephrosis are present in about 30% of fetuses with trisomy 21 and 8% of normal fetuses. Additionally, about 10% of trisomy 21 fetuses may have sonographically detectable anatomical abnormalities such as cardiac anomalies, duodenal atresia, hydrocephalus or hydrops (Benacerraf 1987, Nyberg *et al* 1990). Therefore, the absence of a major abnormality and all four markers would reduce the background risk by about 40% (Table 2.35).

Table 2.35 Maternal age-related risk (1/number in the table) for trisomy 21 at 20 weeks of gestation (background) and in the presence of apparently isolated nuchal fold thickness ≥6 mm (NT) or hyperechogenic bowel (HB) or relatively short femur (SF) or mild hydronephrosis (MH) or a combination of MH and SF. The last column provides an estimate of risks for fetuses with no obvious anatomical abnormalities and none of the four markers.

| Maternal age (yrs) | Background risk | Abnormalities | | | | | No abnormalities |
		NT	HB	SF	MH	MH + SF	
20	1176	63	215	512	784	342	1960
22	1136	61	207	494	758	330	1893
24	1087	58	198	473	725	316	1812
26	990	53	181	431	660	288	1650
28	855	46	156	372	570	249	1425
30	690	37	126	301	460	201	1150
32	508	28	93	221	339	148	847
34	342	19	63	149	228	100	570
36	216	12	40	94	144	63	360
38	129	8	24	57	86	38	215
40	74	5	14	33	50	22	123

The need for caution in the interpretation of results

In the calculation of adjusted risks, we have used the combined data from several studies, but such analysis may not be valid because of the wide variation in findings. For example, the reported prevalence of increased nuchal fold thickening in fetuses with trisomy 21 varied from 16% to 75% and in controls it varied from 0.3% to 3%. Using the average prevalences for the two groups, we calculated that the likelihood ratio for trisomy 21 in the presence of increased nuchal fold thickness is 48. This may be a gross underestimate when the true prevalences are similar to those reported by Benacerraf *et al* (1987) who first described this sonographic marker; the likelihood ratio from their study is 430. Alternatively, it would be a gross overestimate if the true prevalences were well reflected by findings from a large multicentre study that evaluated the marker in routine clinical practice; the likelihood ratio from this study is 10 (Grandjean *et al* 1995).

There are at least four explanations for the large differences between the available data sets. First, criteria for diagnosis of the various sonographic markers have not been standardised. Second, there were differences between the studies in the gestation at which examination took place and, as shown in the previous sections of this chapter, the prevalence of trisomy changes with gestation, being much higher at 16 than 24 weeks. Third, some studies were performed in specialist centres which had a large proportion of high risk or referred pregnancies and probably a higher standard of ultrasound scanning. Finally, data were collected at different ends of a 10-year period during which both the quality of ultrasound equipment and the standard of scanning have improved.

The risk estimates need to be validated by prospective multicentre studies in which the targets of ultrasound examination are clearly defined, i.e. criteria for diagnosis of subtle markers are unified and there is a list of anatomical and biometrical abnormalities for which sonographers specifically look. In such studies, it is necessary to ensure that the sonographers have the skills and equipment that allow diagnosis of markers and anatomical abnormalities and that examination takes place in a small gestational range bracket.

SEQUENTIAL SCREENING

Screening for trisomy 21 by fetal nuchal translucency thickness at 10-14 weeks of gestation and maternal age may identify 80% of affected pregnancies for a false positive rate of 5%. Screening by maternal serum biochemistry at 15-18 weeks and maternal age may identify up to 70% of affected pregnancies for a false positive rate of 5%. As suggested in the previous section, screening by ultrasound examination at around 20 weeks may identify about 40% of affected pregnancies with a false positive rate of about 8%.

Ultrasound scanning for nuchal translucency thickness is likely to become the main method of screening because it has the highest sensitivity, but also because first trimester scanning will inevitably become an inherent part of routine antenatal care for (i) pregnancy dating and viability, (ii) diagnosis of multiple pregnancies and determination of chorionicity, and (iii) early detection of a wide range of fetal abnormalities.

Second trimester biochemical screening has been introduced widely. This method of screening is dependent on accurate dating of the pregnancy and will inevitably depend on the results of a prior ultrasound scan. Even if biochemical screening is proven not to have a major additional (to nuchal translucency screening) beneficial effect in terms of sensitivity for trisomy 21, it is unlikely that this method will be abandoned in the near future. This has certainly been true for maternal serum AFP screening for neural tube defects; although it has been well established for nearly one decade that second trimester ultrasound scanning can identify the vast majority of neural tube defects, many centres are still using AFP screening that can at most identify 80% of such defects.

An ultrasound scan at around 20 weeks of gestation is now offered routinely to all women in most developed countries. With inevitable widespread improvement in the standard of scanning and the quality of equipment, many structural abnormalities and markers of chromosomal defects will be detected and, based on the results of published reports, a high proportion of women will be counselled that they are at increased risk of fetal chromosomal abnormalities. Consequently, a high proportion of the population will be subjected to sequential screening by nuchal translucency scanning at 10-13 weeks, biochemical testing at 15-18 weeks and by ultrasound scanning at around 20 weeks.

Sequential screening could result in a major increase in the rate of invasive testing (from a maximum of 5% for one method of screening to a minimum of 18% if all three methods are used), with an increase in procedure-related fetal death and considerable iatrogenic anxiety for the parents as well as the economic cost involved. Despite this cost, such sequential screening will not necessarily achieve a much higher sensitivity in the detection of trisomy 21.

In order to minimise the major disadvantage of sequential screening (increased invasive testing rate), it is necessary to modify the *a priori* risk of each patient because the prevalence of trisomy 21 in a population that has already been subjected to a screening test and selective termination of affected fetuses is obviously less than in a population that is being screened for the first time. The effect of sequential screening on the residual prevalence of trisomy 21 is illustrated in Table 2.36.

The first step in the interpretation of results from sequential screening is to calculate the gestational age-related prevalence of trisomy 21 at the time of screening. For example, a given population that is not subjected to any form of screening and contains 1000 trisomy 21 fetuses at 12 weeks of gestation will contain only 850 such fetuses at 16 weeks, 750 at 20 weeks and 600 at birth (Table 2.36), because the rate of intrauterine lethality of this chromosomal abnormality between 12 and 16 weeks is 15%, between 12 and 20 weeks is 25%, and between 12 weeks and birth is 40%. Therefore, for a 40 year old woman, the estimated risk for trisomy 21 is 1/57 at 12 weeks, 1/67 at 16 weeks, 1/74 at 20 weeks and 1/97 in live births (Appendix B).

Table 2.36 Effect on reduction in prevalence of trisomy 21 at various stages of pregnancy according to the results of screening tests.

	No screening	12 wk scan (80% detection)		16 wk biochem (70% detection)		20 wk scan (40% detection)	
		Screen +ve	Screen -ve	Screen +ve	Screen -ve	Screen +ve	Screen -ve
12 wks	1000	800	200				
16 wks	850		160-200 4.3-5x reduction	595	255		
20 wks	750				225-255 2.9-3.3x reduction	300	450
Birth	600		120-200		205-255	360-450 1.3-1.7x reduction	

The second step is to calculate the residual prevalence of trisomy 21 in a population that has already been subjected to a previous screening test. Since the prevalence changes with gestation because of spontaneous intrauterine death, the extent of reduction in prevalence by screening and subsequent termination of the affected cases will depend on whether screening preferentially identified those fetuses that were destined to die spontaneously. Alternatively, spontaneous lethality is proportionately distributed between the screen positive and screen negative group.

When a population containing 1000 trisomy 21 fetuses at 12 weeks of gestation is subjected to nuchal translucency screening (which identifies 80% of affected fetuses and in all such cases the parents chose to have termination of pregnancy), the residual number of trisomy 21 fetuses is reduced to 200. It is possible that all 200 such fetuses would be alive at 16 weeks because increased translucency at 12 weeks had preferentially detected all of the cases that would have died spontaneously between 12 and 16 weeks. Therefore, the prevalence of trisomy 21 at 16 weeks would have been reduced from the expected 850 (if there was no previous screening) to 200 which is equivalent to a 4.3-fold decrease. Alternatively, if the rate of intrauterine lethality was the same in both groups, then 170 trisomy 21 fetuses would still be alive at 16 weeks, which would then represent a 5-fold reduction (170/850) in the prevalence of trisomy 21 at 16 weeks. Based on these calculations, the prevalence of trisomy 21 at birth would be 120–200, rather than 600 in a population that did not have antenatal screening.

This methodology has also been applied to determine that, in a patient with a screen negative result after biochemical screening at 16 weeks, at the time of the 20-week scan the risk for trisomy 21 is reduced by a factor of 2.9–3.3 and the prevalence is 225–255, rather than 750 in a population that did not have biochemical screening. Consequently, the prevalence at birth would be 205–255, rather than 600. Screening by a 20-week ultrasound scan would be associated with a 1.3–1.7 fold reduction in the prevalence of trisomy 21 at birth from 600 to between 360 and 450 (Table 2.36).

Calculation of individual risks

For a given patient, the estimated risk for trisomy 21 after a screening test can be adjusted according to the likelihood ratio of a previous screening test. For example, in a 40-year-old woman at 16 weeks of gestation, the maternal age-related risk for trisomy 21 is 1/67. She had biochemical testing at 16 weeks which reduced her risk to 1/130. She also had first trimester nuchal translucency screening that had reduced her age-related risk by a factor of 3.5. Therefore, the new estimated risk for trisomy 21 after biochemical screening can be reduced by this factor of 3.5 to become 1/455.

This proposal is based on the assumption that those trisomic pregnancies with increased fetal nuchal translucency thickness are not more likely to be the very ones with abnormal maternal serum biochemistry at 15–18 weeks. Brizot *et al* (1994) have shown that, certainly in the first trimester, there is no significant association between translucency thickness and maternal serum PAPP-A or hCG and it is reasonable to assume that the same may be true for second trimester serum markers.

Similarly, the proposal assumes that pregnancies with abnormal serum biochemistry are not more likely to be the ones with sonographic markers at 20 weeks of gestation. Since trisomic pregnancies with increased first trimester nuchal translucency may well be the very ones with certain abnormal second trimester sonographic markers, such as cardiac defects or increased nuchal fold thickness, it is best that, at present, those with a screen negative result from the nuchal translucency scan should not have their risk further reduced by a negative second trimester scan.

REFERENCES

Achiron R, Barkai G, Katznelson MBM, Mashiach S. Fetal lateral ventricle choroid plexus cysts: the dilemma of amniocentesis. Obstet Gynecol 1991;78:815-18.

Antonarakis SE, Lewi JG, Adelsberger PA, Petersen MB, Schinzel AA, Cohen MM, Roulston D, Schwartz S, Mikkelsen M, Tranebjorg L, Greenberg F, How DI, Rudd NL. Parental origin of the extra chromosome in Trisomy 21 as indicated by analysis of DNA polymorphisms. N Engl J Med 1991;324:872-6.

Benacerraf BR, Gelman R, Frigoletto FD. Sonographic identification of second-trimester fetuses with Down's syndrome. N Engl J Med 1987;317:1371-6.

Benacerraf, BR, Harlow B, Frigoletto FD. Are choroid plexus cysts an indication for second trimester amniocentesis? Am J Obstet Gynecol 1990a;162:1001-6.

Benacerraf BR, Mandell J, Estroff JA, Harlow BL, Frigoletto FD. Fetal pyelectasis: a possible association with Down syndrome. Obstet Gynecol 1990b;76:58-60.

Benacerraf BR, Nadel A, Bromley B. Identification of second-trimester fetuses with autosomal trisomy by use of a sonographic scoring index. Radiology 1994;193:135-40.

Bleyer A. Indication that mongoloid imbecility is a gametogenic mutation of degenerating type. Am J Dis Child 1934;47:342.

Boyers SP, Diamond MP, Lavy G, Russell JB, DeCherney AH. The effect of polyploidy on embryo cleavage after in vitro fertilization in humans. Fertil Steril 1987;48:624-7.

Brizot ML, Snijders RJM, Bersinger NA, Kuhn P, Nicolaides KH. Maternal serum pregnancy-associated plasma protein A and fetal nuchal translucency thickness for the prediction of fetal trisomies in early pregnancy. Obstet Gynecol 1994;84:918–22.

Brizot ML, Snijders RJM, Butler J, Bersinger NA, Nicolaides KH. Maternal serum hCG and fetal nuchal translucency thickness in the prediction of fetal trisomies in the first trimester of pregnancy. Br J Obstet Gynaecol 1995;102: 127–32.

Bromley B, Doubilet P, Frigoletto FD, Krauss C, Estroff JA, Benacerraf BR. Is fetal hyperechogenic bowel on second-trimester sonogram an indication for amniocentesis? Obstet Gynecol 1994;83:647-51.

Calzolari E, Volpato S, Bianchi F, Cianciulli D, Tenconi R, Clementi M, Calabro A, Lungarotti S, Mastroiacovo PP, Botto L *et al*. Omphalocele and gastroschisis: a collaborative study of five Italian congenital malformation registries. Teratology 1993;47:47-55.

Carpenter MW, Curci MR, Dibbens AW, Haddow JE. Perinatal management of ventral wall defects. Obstet Gynecol 1984;64:646.

Carr DH. Chromosome studies in abortuses and stillborn infants. Lancet 1963;2:603-6.

Chan L, Hixson JL, Laifer SA, Marchese SG, Martin JG, Hill LM. A sonographic and karyotypic study of second trimester fetal choroid plexus cysts. Obstet Gynecol 1989;73:703-5.

Chinn DH, Miller EI, Worthy LM, Towers CV. Sonographically detected fetal choroid plexus cysts: frequency and association with aneuploidy. J Ultrasound Med 1991;10:255-8.

Chitkara U, Cogswell C, Norton K, Wilkins IA. Choroid plexus cysts in the fetus: a benign anatomic variant or pathological entity? Obstet Gynecol 1988;72:185-9.

Chitty LS, Hunt GH, Moore J, Lobb MO. Effectiveness of routine ultrasonography in detecting fetal structural abnormalities in a low risk population. Br Med J 1991;303:1165-9.

Chudleigh P, Pearce JM, Campbell S. The prenatal diagnosis of transient cysts of the fetal choroid plexus. Prenat Diagn 1984;4:135-7.

Clark SL, De Vore GR, Sabey PL. Prenatal diagnosis of cysts of the fetal choroid plexus. Obstet Gynecol 1988;72:585-7.

Corteville JE, Dicke JM, Crane JP. Fetal pyelectasis and Down syndrome: is genetic amniocentesis warranted? Obstet Gynecol 1992;79:770-2.

Crane JP, Gray DL. Sonographically measured nuchal skinfold thickness as a screening tool for Down syndrome: results of a prospective clinical trial. Obstet Gynecol 1991;77:533-6.

Cuckle HS, Wald NJ, Thompson SG. Estimating a woman's risk of having a pregnancy associated with Down's syndrome using her age and serum alpha-fetoprotein level. Br J Obstet Gynaecol 1987;94:387-402.

Cuckle H, Wald N, Quinn J, Royston P, Butler L. Ultrasound fetal femur length measurement in the screening for Down's syndrome. Br J Obstet Gynaecol 1989;96:1373-8.

DeRoo TR, Harris RD, Sargent SK, Denholm TA, Crow HC. Fetal choroid plexus cysts: prevalence, clinical significance and sonographic appearence. Am J Roentgenol 1988;151:1179-81.

DeVore GR, Alfi O. The association between an abnormal nuchal skin fold, trisomy 21, and ultrasound abnormalities during the second trimester of pregnancy. Ultrasound Obstet Gynecol 1993;3:387-94.

Dicke JM, Gray DL, Songster GS, Crane JP. Fetal biometry as a screening tool for the detection of chromosomally abnormal pregnancies. Obstet Gynecol 1989;74:726-9.

Dicke JM, Crane JP. Sonographically detected hyperechogenic fetal bowel: significance and implications for pregnancy management. Obstet. Gynecol 1992;80:778-82.

Down JLH. Observations on an ethnic classification of idiots. Clinical Lecture Reports, London Hospital 1866;3:259.

Edwards JH. A new trisomic syndrome. Lancet 1960;i:787.

Ferguson-Smith MA, Yates JRW. Maternal age specific rates for chromosomal aberrations and factors influencing them: report of a collaborative European study on 52,965 amniocenteses. Prenat Diagn 1984;4:5-44.

Fraser J, Mitchell A. Kalmuk idiocy. Report of a case with autopsy. J Ment Sci 1876;98:169-79.

Ginsberg N, Cadkin A, Pergament E, Verlinsky V. Ultrasonographic detection of the second-trimester fetus with trisomy 18 and trisomy 21. Am J Obstet Gynecol 1990;163:1186-90.

Grandjean H, Sarramon MF, AFDPHE Study Group. Sonographic measurement of nuchal fold thickness for detection of Down syndrome in the second-trimester fetus: a multicentre study. Obstet Gynecol 1995;85:103-6.

Hasan S, Hermansen MC. The prenatal diagnosis of ventral abdominal wall defects. Am J Obstet Gynecol 1986;155:842.

Hecht CA, Hook EB. The imprecision in rates of Down syndrome by 1-year maternal age intervals: a critical analysis of rates used in biochemical screening. Prenat Diagn 1994;14:729-38.

Hill LM, Guzick D, Belfar HL, Hixson J, Rivello D, Rusnak J. The current role of sonography in the detection of Down syndrome. Obstet Gynecol 1989;74:620-3.

Hook EB, Chambers GM. Estimates of rates of Down syndrome in live births by one year maternal age intervals for mothers aged 20-49 in a New York State study. In: Bergsma D, Lowry RB, Trimble BK, Feingold M 1977 (Eds.) Numerical taxonomy of birth defects and polygenic disorders, Birth Defects Original Article Series Vol 13, No 3A, New York: Alan R. Liss.

Hook EB, Fabia JJ. Frequency of Down syndrome in livebirths by single-year maternal age interval: results of a Massachusetts study. Teratology 1978;17:223-8.

Hook EB, Lindsjo A. Down syndrome in live births by single year maternal age interval in a Swedish study: comparison with results from a New York State study. Am J Hum Genet 1978;30:19-27.

Hook EB, Woodbury DF, Albright SG. Rates of trisomy 18 in livebirths, stillbirths, and at amniocentesis. Birth Defects 1979;15:81-93.

Hook EB. Rates of 47, + 13 amd 46 translocation D/13 Patau syndrome in live births and comparison with rates in fetal deaths and at amniocentesis. Am J Hum Genet 1980;32:849-58.

Hook EB. Chromosome abnormalities and spontaneous fetal death following amniocentesis: further data and associations with maternal age. Am J Hum Genet 1983;35:110-16.

Hook EB, Cross PK, Regal RR. The frequency of 47,+21, 47,+18, and 47,+13 at the uppermost extremes of maternal ages: results on 56,094 fetuses studied prenatally and comparisons with data on livebirths. Hum Genet 1984; 68:211-20.

Howard RJ, Tuck SM, Long J, Thomas VA. The significance of choroid plexus cysts in fetuses at 18-20 weeks. An indication for amniocentesis? Prenat Diagn 1992;12:685-8.

Hsu LYF, Kaffe S, Jenkins EC, Alonso C, Benn PA, David K, Hirschhorn K, Lieber E, Shanska A, Shapino LR, Schutta E, Warburton D. Proposed guidelines for diagnosis of chromosome mosaicism in amniocytes based on data derived from chromosome mosaicism and pseudomosaicism studies. Prenat Diag 1992;12:555-73.

Huether CA, Gummere GR, Hook EB. Down's syndrome: percentage reporting on birth certificates and single year maternal age risk for Ohio 1970-79: comparison with upstate New York data. Am J Public Health 1981;71:1367-72.

Kirk EP, Wah RM. Obstetric management of the fetus with omphalocele or gastroschisis. Am J Obstet Gynecol 1983;146:512.

Kirk JS, Comstock CH, Fassnacht MA. Routine measurement of nuchal thickness in the second trimester. J Maternal-Fetal Medicine 1992;1:82-6.

Koulisher L, Gillerot Y. Down's syndrome in Wallonia (South Belgium), 1971-1978: cytogenetics and incidence. Hum Genet 1980;54:243-50.

Levi S, Hyjazi Y, Schaaps JP, Defoort P, Colon R, Buekens P. Sensitivity and specificity of routine antenatal screening for congenital anomalies by ultrasound: The Belgian multi-centric study. Ultrasound Obstet Gynecol 1991;1:102-10.

Lockwood C, Benacerraf B, Krinsky A, Blakemore K, Belanger K, Mahoney M, Hobbins J. A sonographic screening method for Down syndrome. Am J Obstet Gynecol 1987;157:803-8.

Mabogunje OOA, Mahour GH. Omphalocele and gastroschisis: trends in survival across two decades. Am J Surg 1984;148:679-86.

Nicolaides KH, Rodeck CH, Gosden CM. Rapid karyotyping in non-lethal fetal abnormalities. Lancet 1986;I:283-7.

Nicolaides KH, Snijders RJM, Gosden CM, Berry C, Campbell S. Ultrasonographically detectable markers of fetal chromosomal abnormalities. Lancet 1992a;340:704-7.

Nicolaides KH, Cheng HH, Abbas A, Snijders RJ, Gosden C. Fetal renal defects: associated malformations and chromosomal defects. Fetal Diagn Ther 1992b;7:1-11.

Nyberg DA, Resta RG, Luthy DA, Hickok DE, Mahony BS, Hirsch JH. Prenatal sonographic findings of Down syndrome: review of 94 cases. Obstet Gynecol 1990;76:370-7.

Nyberg DA, Kramer D, Resta RG, Kapur R. Prenatal sonographic findings of trisomy 18. J Ultrasound Med 1993;2:103-13.

Nyberg DA, Resta RG, Luthy DA, Hickok DE, Williams MS. Humerus and femur length shortening in the detection of Down's syndrome. Am J Obstet Gynecol 1993c;168:534-8.

Nyberg DA, Resta RG, Mahony BS, Dubinsky T, Luthy DA, Hickok DE, Luthardt FW. Fetal hyperechogenic bowel and Down's syndrome. Ultrasound Obstet Gynecol 1993b;3:330-3.

Ostlere SJ, Irving HC, Lilford RJ. Fetal choroid plexus cysts: a report of 100 cases. Radiology 1990;175:753-5.

Patau K, Smith DW, Therman E, Inhorn SL, Wagnes HP. Multiple congenital anomaly caused by an extra chromosome. Lancet 1960;1:790-3.

Perpignano MC, Cohen HL, Klein VR, Mandel FS, Streltzoff J, Chervenak FA, Goldman MA. Fetal choroid plexus cysts: beware the smaller cyst. Radiology 1992;182:715-17.

Platt LD, Carlson DE, Medeans AL. Fetal choroid plexus cysts in the second trimester, a cause for concern. Am J Obstet Gynecol 1991;164:1652-6.

Porto M, Murata Y, Warneke LA, Keegan KA Jr. Fetal choroid plexus cysts: an independent risk factor for chromosomal anomalies. J Clin Ultrasound 1993;21:103-8.

Rodis JF, Vintzileos AM, Fleming AD, Ciarlegio L, Nardi DA, Feeney L, Scorza WE, Campbell WA, Ingardia C. Comparison of humerus length with femur length in fetuses with Down syndrome. Am J Obstet Gynecol 1991;165:1051-6.

Schreinemachers DM, Cross PK, Hook EB. Rates of trisomies 21, 18, 13 and other chromosome abnormalities in about 20,000 prenatal studies compared with estimated rates in live births. Hum Genet 1982;61:318-24.

Scioscia AL, Pretorius DH, Budorick NE, Cahill TC, Axelrod FT, Leopold GR. Second-trimester echogenic bowel and chromosomal abnormalities. Am J Obstet Gynecol 1992;167:889-94.

Shuttleworth GE. Mongoloid imbecility. Br Med J 1909;2:661-5.

Snijders RJM, Sebire NJ, Nicolaides KH. Maternal age and gestational age-specific risk for chromosomal defects. Fetal Diag Ther 1995a (in press).

Snijders RJM, Sebire NJ, Faria M, Patel F, Nicolaides KH. Fetal mild hydronephrosis and chromosomal defects: relation to maternal age and gestation. Fetal Diag Ther 1995b (in press).

Snijders RJM, Sebire NJ, Souka A, Santiago C, Nicolaides KH. Fetal exomphalos and chromosomal defects: relation to maternal age and gestation. Ultrasound Obstet Gynecol 1995c (in press).

Snijders RJM, Sebire NJ, Psarra A, Souka A, Nicolaides KH. Prevalence of fetal facial cleft at different stages of pregnancy. Ultrasound Obstet Gynecol 1995d (in press)

Snijders RJM, Shawwa L, Nicolaides KH. Fetal choroid plexus cysts and trisomy 18: assessment of risk based on ultrasound findings and maternal age. Prenat Diagn 1994;14:1119–27.

Sutherland GR, Clisby SR, Bloor G. Down's syndrome in South Australia. Med J Aust 1979;2:58-61.

Tabor A, Philip J, Madsen M, Bang J, Obel EB, Norgaard-Pedersen B. Randomised controlled trial of genetic amniocentesis in 4606 low-risk women. Lancet 1986;1:1287-93.

Trimble BK, Baird PA. Maternal age and Down syndrome: age-specific incidence rates by single year intervals. Am J Med Genet 1978;2:1-5.

Twining P, Zuccollo J, Clewes J, Swallow J. Fetal choroid plexus cysts: a prospective study and review of the literature. Br J Radiol 1991;64:98-102.

Van Zalen-Sprock MM, Van Vugt JM, Karsdorp VH, Maas R, Van Geijn HP. Ultrasound diagnosis of fetal abnormalities and cytogenetic evaluation. Prenat Diagn 1991;11:655-60.

Walkinshaw S, Pilling D, Spriggs A. Isolated choroid plexus cysts - the need for routine offer of karyotyping. Prenat Diagn 1994;14:663-7.

Watson WJ, Miller RC, Menard K, Chescheir NC, Katz VL, Hansen WF. Ultrasonographic measurements of fetal nuchal skin to screen for chromosomal abnormalities. Am J Obstet Gynecol 1994;170:583-6.

Wilson RD, Chitayat D, McGillivray BC. Fetal ultrasound abnormalities: correlation with fetal karyotype, autopsy findings, and postnatal outcome - five-year prospective study. Am J Med Genet 1992;44:586-90.

Wladimiroff JW, Molenaar JC, Niermeijer MF, Stewart PH, van-Eyck J. Prenatal diagnosis and management of omphalocele. Eur J Obstet Gynecol Reprod Biol 1983;16:19.

Young D, Williams EM, Newcombe RG. Down syndrome and maternal age in South Glamorgan. J Med Genet 1980;17:433-6.

First trimester fetal nuchal translucency

OVERVIEW

PREGNANCY DATING
    Crown–rump length in chromosomally normal fetuses
    Crown–rump length in chromosomally abnormal fetuses

ASSESSMENT OF NUCHAL TRANSLUCENCY THICKNESS
    Measurement
    Repeatability

NUCHAL TRANSLUCENCY AND CHROMOSOMAL DEFECTS
    Observational studies
    Screening in high risk populations
    Screening in unselected populations

DEVELOPMENT OF A MODEL FOR SCREENING
    Nuchal translucency
    Nuchal translucency and fetal heart rate
    Nuchal translucency and maternal serum biochemistry

PATHOLOGICAL FINDINGS

EVOLUTION OF NUCHAL TRANSLUCENCY
    Trisomy 21 fetuses
    Chromosomally normal fetuses

NUCHAL TRANSLUCENCY IN MULTIPLE PREGNANCIES

OVERVIEW

Increased nuchal translucency at 10–14 weeks of gestation is a common phenotypic expression of trisomies, Turner syndrome and triploidy (Figure 3.1). This chapter examines the development of a new method of screening for chromosomal defects based on the combination of fetal nuchal translucency thickness, maternal age and maternal serum biochemistry during the first trimester of pregnancy.

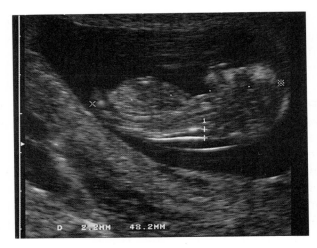

Figure 3.1 Ultrasound picture of fetus at 11 weeks of gestation and nuchal translucency thickness of 2.2 mm. The amnion can be seen as a separate membrane from the fetal skin.

In the 1980s and early 1990s several case reports and small series in high-risk pregnancies demonstrated a possible association between abnormal nuchal fluid and chromosomal defects in the first trimester of pregnancy. Although in some studies the condition was defined as a multiseptated, thin-walled cystic mass similar to that seen in the second trimester, in others the term was used loosely to include nuchal thickening or oedema. We prefer the use of the term translucency because this is the ultrasonographic feature that is observed. Furthermore, increased translucency seen in either chromosomally normal or abnormal fetuses usually resolves during the second trimester; it rarely evolves into nuchal oedema or generalised hydrops.

The first screening studies involved measurement of nuchal translucency thickness immediately before fetal karyotyping for advanced maternal age, parental anxiety, or family history of chromosomal defects in the absence of parental translocations. The frequency of chromosomal defects was examined in relation to both the fetal nuchal translucency thickness and the maternal age distribution of the population. These studies demonstrated that the observed number of trisomies 21, 18 or 13 in fetuses with translucency less than 2.5 mm (or 3 mm for machines that do not give decimals) was approximately five times less than the number expected on the basis of maternal age, whereas for translucencies of $\geq$2.5 mm there was a 12-fold increase in risk. In subsequent studies of more than 1,000 fetuses with translucency of $\geq$2.5 mm, it was possible to derive risks for trisomies with increasing translucency thickness; thus translucencies of 3 mm, 4 mm, 5 mm and $\geq$5.5 mm were associated with three-fold, 18-fold, 28-fold and 36-fold increases in maternal age-related risks.

Subsequently, screening studies of unselected populations were carried out. These studies established the distribution of nuchal translucency thickness with crown–rump length in chromosomally normal and abnormal fetuses and from the overlapping distributions it was possible to calculate risks for chromosomal defects with any given nuchal translucency thickness. Such studies also established that the risks for trisomies can be derived by combining data from maternal age, fetal nuchal translucency thickness, fetal heart rate and maternal serum concentrations of placental products.

PREGNANCY DATING

In 10–45% of pregnancies, women are uncertain of their last menstrual period, they have irregular menstrual cycles or they became pregnant soon after stopping the oral contraceptive pill (Campbell *et al* 1985, Bergsiø *et al* 1990). Additionally, because of considerable variations in the day of ovulation, in approximately 10% of women with certain dates and regular 28-day cycles there is a more than 7-day discrepancy in gestation calculated from the menstrual history and ultrasound (Geirsson 1991). For these reasons accurate dating of pregnancy necessitates ultrasono-graphic examination. This is especially important in screening for chromosomal defects because both the fetal nuchal translucency thickness and the concentration of maternal serum biochemical markers change with gestational age.

In the second and third trimesters of pregnancy intrauterine growth retardation is a common feature of chromosomal defects and, if this is evident from the first trimester, routine pregnancy dating by measurement of crown–rump length will affect the interpretation of results from screening. This section examines whether fetuses with aneuploidies demonstrate evidence of growth retardation during the first trimester.

Crown–rump length in chromosomally normal fetuses

Kuhn *et al* (1995) established a normal range for crown–rump length with gestation (Figure 3.2) from data of 700 chromosomally normal fetuses (25 cases for each gestational day between 70 and 97 days). Ultrasound examinations were

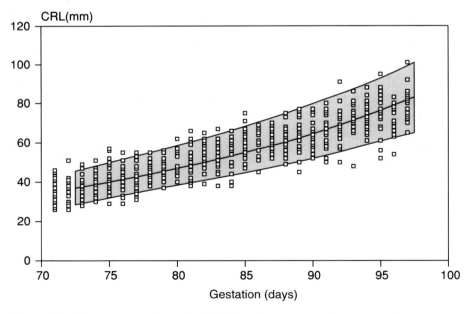

Figure 3.2 Crown–rump length (CRL) in chromosomally normal fetuses. The lines represent the normal range with gestation (mean, 5th and 95th centiles).

performed transabdominally and the crown–rump length was measured on the screen by placing the calipers at the outer edge of the cephalic pole and the outer edge of the fetal rump.The selection criteria were (i) known last menstrual period with a cycle length of 26–30 days, (ii) no history of pregnancy or use of oral contraceptives in the 3-month period before conception, (iii) ultrasonographic examination at 70–97 days since the first day of the last menstrual period, and (iv) live birth of healthy infants at term with birth weight between the 3rd and 97th centiles of the normal range.

Crown–rump length in chromosomally abnormal fetuses

In 135 fetuses with chromosomal defects the median crown–rump length in fetuses with trisomies 21 and 13 or sex chromosome aneuploidies was not significantly different from normal, whereas in trisomy 18 there was evidence of early onset intrauterine growth retardation (Kuhn *et al* 1995).

These findings were confirmed in an extended series of 200 fetuses with chromosomal defects examined at the Harris Birthright Research Centre for Fetal Medicine (Figures 3.3, 3.4 and 3.5; Table 3.1). Similarly, in three other studies involving a total of 154 fetuses with trisomy 21, the crown–rump length was not significantly different from normal and in two studies on a total of 37 fetuses with trisomy 18 the crown–rump length was decreased (Lynch and Berkowitz 1989, Drugan *et al* 1992, Wald *et al* 1993).

These findings suggest that a policy of routine pregnancy dating by measurement of crown–rump length will not affect the interpretation of results from nuchal translucency or biochemical

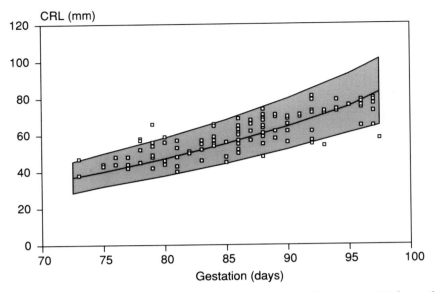

Figure 3.3 Crown–rump length (CRL) in 111 fetuses with trisomy 21 from the Harris Birthright Research Centre for Fetal Medicine, plotted on the normal range with gestation (mean, 5th and 95th centiles).

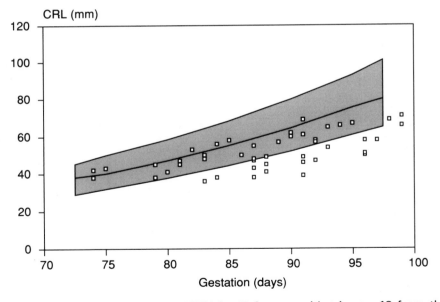

Figure 3.4 Crown–rump length (CRL) in 49 fetuses with trisomy 18 from the Harris Birthright Research Centre for Fetal Medicine, plotted on the normal range with gestation (mean, 5th and 95th centiles).

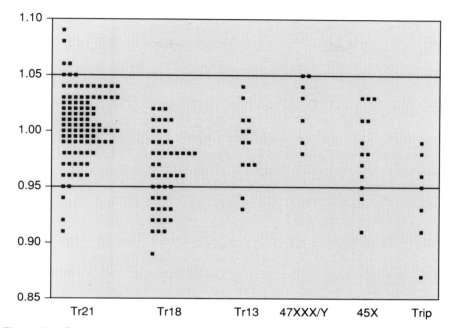

Figure 3.5 Crown–rump length in 200 chromosomally abnormal fetuses seen at the Harris Birthright Research Centre for Fetal Medicine. The individual values are expressed as multiples of the normal median (MoM) for gestation. The horizontal lines represent the normal 5th and 95th centiles.

Table 3.1 Median crown–rump length (CRL) of 200 chromosomally abnormal fetuses diagnosed at the Harris Birthright Centre for Fetal Medicine. The individual values are expressed as multiples of the normal median (MoM) for gestation.

Chromosomal defect	N	CRL in MoM (Range)	p
Trisomy 21	111	1.00 (0.89-1.11)	ns
Trisomy 18	49	0.96 (0.89-1.02)	$p<0.0001$
Trisomy 13	13	0.98 (0.97-1.01)	ns
47,XXX/XXY	7	1.03 (0.98-1.05)	ns
Turner syndrome	13	0.98 (0.91-1.03)	ns
Triploidy	7	0.95 (0.85-0.99)	$p<0.05$

screening since the crown–rump length in fetuses with most chromosomal defects is not different from normal. Although a policy of dating by ultrasound could miss early onset growth retardation due to trisomy 18 or triploidy, the majority of such fetuses will be identified by the presence of a large translucency.

ASSESSMENT OF NUCHAL TRANSLUCENCY THICKNESS

Measurement

Transabdominal ultrasound examination is performed to obtain a sagittal section of the fetus for measurement of fetal crown–rump length. The maximum thickness of the subcutaneous translucency between the skin and the soft tissue overlying the cervical spine is measured (Nicolaides *et al* 1992). Care is taken to distinguish between fetal skin and amnion because at this gestation both structures appear as thin membranes (Figure 3.1). This is achieved by waiting for spontaneous fetal movement away from the amniotic membrane; alternatively, the fetus is bounced off the amnion by asking the mother to cough and/or by tapping the maternal abdomen. All sonographers performing fetal scans should be capable of measuring reliably the crown–rump length and obtaining a proper sagittal view of the fetal spine. For such sonographers it is easy to acquire, within a few hours, the skill to measure accurately nuchal translucency thickness.

Repeatability

A potential criticism of screening by ultrasound, in contrast to biochemical testing, is that scanning requires not only highly skilled operators but it is also prone to operator variability.

In a prospective study to assess the repeatability of measurement of fetal nuchal translucency thickness at 10–14 weeks of gestation, the translucency was measured by two of four operators in 200 pregnant women (Pandya *et al* 1995a). To assess repeatability of different components of variability, six measurements of nuchal translucency were made on each fetus. The first operator generated the appropriate image and measured the translucency and then generated a new image and repeated the measurement (intra-observer repeatability). This second image was frozen on the screen but the calipers were removed and the second operator reset the calipers and made a measurement (caliper placement repeatability). The process was then repeated with the operators reversed (inter-observer repeatability).This study demonstrated that, when the nuchal translucency thickness is measured by well trained operators, the measurement is highly reproducible (Figure 3.6). The repeatability was unrelated to the size of the nuchal translucency and, when the mean of two measurements was used, 95% of the time the intra-observer and inter-observer repeatabilities were 0.54 mm and 0.62 mm, respectively.

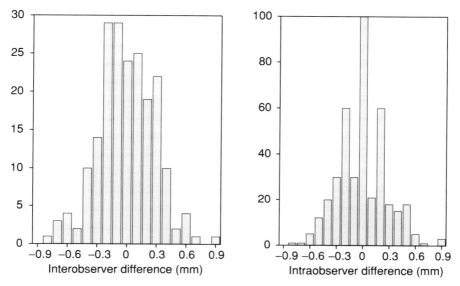

Figure 3.6 Frequency distribution of differences between measurements by two observers (left) and of differences between repeated measurements by the same observer (right).

The difference in repeat readings by the same observer and between observers may be accounted for by two main factors. Firstly, the generation of a new image during which the fetal position may have changed by flexion or extension of the fetal neck and by rotation of the spine to the anterior or posterior position, and second, the correct placement of the calipers. In this study the caliper placement repeatability was similar to the intra-observer and inter-observer repeatability, suggesting that a large part of the variation in measurements can be accounted for by the placement of the calipers rather than the generation of the image. Digital image processing and automation of caliper placement should reduce the differences in repeatability. In the meantime, it is best to take the mean of two good measurements rather than one.

NUCHAL TRANSLUCENCY AND CHROMOSOMAL DEFECTS

Observational studies

Several studies documented a strong association between abnormal nuchal translucency and chromosomal defects (Table 3.2).

Table 3.2 Summary of reported series on first trimester fetal nuchal translucency providing data on gestational age (GA), criteria for diagnosis (C) and the presence of associated chromosomal defects. In some series the translucency is merely referred to as cystic hygroma (CH) and no data on thickness are given. 21=trisomy 21, 18=trisomy 18, 13=trisomy 13, Oth=other

Author	GA (wks)	C	N	Chromosomal defect					
				Total	21	18	13	45X	Oth
Gustavii et al 84	12	CH	1	0%	-	-	-	-	-
Dallapicolla et al 84	12	CH	1	0%	-	-	-	-	-
Reuss et al 87a,87b	10-12	CH	2	50%	-	-	-	1	-
Cohen et al 89	12	CH	1	100%	-	1	-	-	-
Pons et al 89	11-14	CH	4	100%	1	3	-	1	-
Rottem et al 89	10	CH	1	100%	1	-	-	-	-
Bronshtein et al 89	11-12	CH	2	50%	-	-	-	-	-
Hill et al 91	13-14	CH	2	100%	-	2	-	-	-
MacLeod et al 91	10-14	CH	5	90%	-	1	1	2	-
Sepulveda & Giaffardi 92	11	CH	2	50%	-	-	-	1	-
Johnson et al 93	10-14	≥2.0	68	60%	16	9	2	9	5
Hewitt et al 93	10-14	≥2.0	29	41%	5	3	1	2	1
Shulman et al 92	10-13	≥2.5	32	47%	4	4	3	4	-
Nicolaides et al 92,94b	10-13	≥3.0	88	38%	21	8	2	-	2
Pandya et al 94,95d	10-13	≥3.0	1015	19%	101	51	13	14	15
Szabo & Gellen 90	11-12	≥3.0	8	88%	7	-	-	-	-
Wilson et al 92	8-11	≥3.0	14	21%	-	-	-	1	2
Ville et al 92	9-14	≥3.0	29	28%	4	3	1	-	-
Trauffer et al 94	10-14	≥3.0	43	49%	9	4	1	4	3
Brambati et al 95	8-15	≥3.0	70	19%	?	?	?	?	?
Comas et al 95	9-13	≥3.0	51	18%	4	4	-	-	1
Nadel et al 93	10-15	≥4.0	63	68%	15	15	1	10	2
Savoldelli et al 93	9-12	≥4.0	24	79%	15	2	1	1	-
Schulte-Valentin 92	10-14	≥4.0	8	88%	7	-	-	-	-
van Zalen-Sprock 92	10-14	≥4.0	18	28%	3	1	-	1	1
Cullen et al 90	11-13	≥6.0	29	52%	6	2	-	4	3
Suchet et al 92	8-14	≥10	13	62%	-	-	-	7	1
Total	**8-15**		**1623**	**29%**	**219**	**113**	**26**	**62**	**36**

Although the mean frequency of chromosomal defects in 30 series involving a total of 1,593 patients was 29%, there were large differences between the studies with the frequency ranging from 0% to 100%. This variation in results was presumably the consequence of both the failure to take into account the maternal age distribution of the populations examined, and differences in the definition of minimum thickness of the abnormal translucency (undefined in the early studies and ranging from 2 mm to 10 mm in the later ones).

Screening in high risk populations

In a prospective study of 827 women with singleton pregnancies undergoing first trimester fetal karyotyping because of advanced maternal age, parental anxiety or a family history of a chromosomal abnormality in the absence of balanced parental translocation, the translucency thickness was measured (Nicolaides *et al* 1992). This study suggested that invasive testing for patients with translucency of ≥2.5 mm or ≥3.5 mm would identify 80% and 70%, respectively of trisomic fetuses with corresponding false positive rates of 4.1% and 1.1%. In an expanded series of 1,273 pregnancies, trisomies 21, 18 or 13 were found in 2.8% of the cases (Nicolaides *et al* 1994b). The translucency thickness was ≥2.5 mm in 86.1% of the trisomic and in 4.5% of the chromosomally normal fetuses (Table 3.3).

Table 3.3 Translucency thickness and fetal karyotype (Nicolaides *et al* 1994b).

Nuchal thickness	N	Fetal karyotype				
		Normal	Abnormal			
			Tr 21	Tr 18	Tr 13	Other*
<3 mm	1,185	1,172	4	1	-	8
3 mm	52	43	6	-	1	2
4 mm	14	6	5	2	1	-
5 mm	10	2	7	1	-	-
>5 mm	12	4	3	5	-	-
Total	**1,273**	**1,227**	**25**	**9**	**2**	**10**

* 46,XX ,18p-; 47,XXX (n=2); 47,XXY (n=2); 47,XXX/46,XX; 47,XX+21/46,XX; 47,XX+8/46,XX; 47,XX+22; 47,XY+fragment.

In the group with normal fetal karyotype, the incidence of nuchal translucency ≥2.5 mm was independent of maternal age and it was therefore possible to derive estimates of risks for fetal trisomies on the basis of maternal age and fetal nuchal translucency thickness; translucency of less than 2.5 mm was associated with a 4.5-fold reduction, whereas translucency of ≥2.5 mm was associated with 12-fold increase in maternal age-related risk (Nicolaides *et al* 1994b).

In a study of 560 pregnancies with increased fetal nuchal translucency thickness (2.5–9 mm) at 10–14 weeks of gestation, fetal karyotyping was performed (Pandya *et al* 1994). The incidence of chromosomal defects increased with both maternal age and translucency thickness. In an expanded series of 1,015 pregnancies with increased fetal nuchal translucency thickness, 193 (19%) were associated with chromosomal defects (Table 3.4; Pandya *et al* 1995d).

Table 3.4 Fetal nuchal translucency thickness and frequency of chromosomal abnormalities in 1,015 fetuses with a minimum translucency of 2.5 mm (Pandya *et al* 1995d).

Nuchal thickness	N	Abnormal karyotype					
		Total	Trisomies			Sex chromosomes		Other*
			21	18	13	45,X	47,XXY/XXY	
3 mm	696	7%	24	8	2	1	4	11
4 mm	139	27%	26	5	3	-	-	4
5 mm	66	53%	24	8	2	-	-	1
6 mm	39	49%	6	9	1	3	-	-
7 mm	24	83%	6	10	1	3	-	-
8 mm	23	70%	6	6	3	1	-	-
9 mm	28	78%	8	5	1	6	-	-
Total	1,015	19%	101	51	13	14	4	16

* Triploidy (n=10), 47,XY+fr; 47,XX+22; 46,XX-4p; 46,XYm16; 47,XY+20; 47,XX+22

The observed number of trisomies 21, 18 and 13 in fetuses with translucencies of 3 mm, 4 mm, 5 mm, and ≥6 mm was approximately three times, 18 times, 28 times and 36 times higher than the respective number expected on the basis of maternal age (Table 3.5; Figure 3.7). The incidences of Turner syndrome and triploidy were nine times and eight times higher but the incidence of other sex chromosome aneuploidies was similar to that expected (Pandya *et al* 1995d).

Table 3.5 Observed number of trisomies 21, 18 and 13 in relation to fetal nuchal translucency thickness and the expected number on the basis of maternal age (Pandya *et al* 1995d).

Nuchal thickness	N	Observed		Expected		Observed to expected ratio	
		21	18 &13	21	18 &13	21	18 &13
3 mm	696	24	10	7.47	3.23	3.2	3.1
4 mm	139	26	8	1.31	0.56	19.8	14.0
5 mm	66	24	10	0.84	0.36	28.6	27.8
≥6 mm	114	26	36	1.20	0.52	21.7	69.2
Total	1,015	100	64	10.82	4.67	9.2	13.7

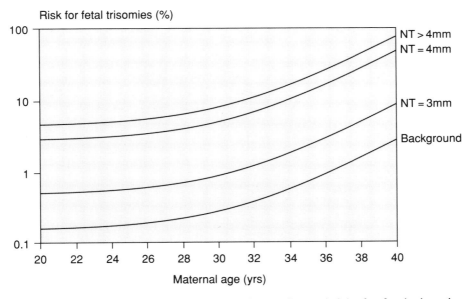

Figure 3.7 Semilogarithmic graph illustrating estimated risks for fetal trisomies 21, 18 or 13 at 10–14 weeks of gestation on the basis of maternal age alone (background) and maternal age with fetal nuchal translucency thickness of 3 mm, 4 mm and >4 mm (Pandya *et al* 1995d).

Screening in unselected populations

The Frimley Park and St Peter's study

Frimley Park and St Peter's are general hospitals within the NHS with a combined annual number of deliveries of approximately 6,000. Prior to the introduction of nuchal translucency scanning, the policy of these hospitals was to offer amniocentesis to women aged 35 years or older. During 1993 there were 11 fetuses with Down's syndrome and only two of these were detected prenatally.

Subsequently, nuchal translucency screening was introduced and the implementation of this policy was achieved without the need for increasing the number of staff or the equipment. Women with fetal translucency of 2.5 mm or more were offered fetal karyotyping. In addition, women aged 35 years or older were offered amniocentesis at 16 weeks' gestation.

The data of the first 5 months after the introduction of the new policy were analysed following completion of the pregnancies (Pandya *et al* 1995b). During this period, 74% of women delivering in the two hospitals attended for first trimester scanning and the nuchal translucency was successfully measured in all pregnancies. The translucency was raised in 3.6% of cases and the total percentage of invasive procedures was 5.1%. All four cases of Down's syndrome that occurred in this period were diagnosed prenatally.

The multi-centre study

In an ongoing study coordinated by the Harris Birthright Research Centre for Fetal Medicine, pregnant women living in London and the surrounding areas are offered ultrasound examination at 10–14 weeks of gestation. The fetal crown–rump length and the nuchal translucency thickness are measured and, when the translucency is $\geq$2.5 mm, the parents are offered the option of fetal karyotyping by chorion villus sampling. The fetal nuchal translucency was $\geq$2.5 mm in 5% of the population and this group included 77% of the 86 cases with trisomy 21 and 78% of the 78 cases with other chromosomal defects (Pandya *et al* 1990).

DEVELOPMENT OF A MODEL FOR SCREENING

Nuchal translucency

Data from the multi-centre study coordinated by the Harris Birthright Research Centre showed that in normal pregnancies the fetal nuchal translucency thickness increases with crown–rump length and that in pregnancies with chromosomally abnormal fetuses measurements are relatively high (Figure 3.8).

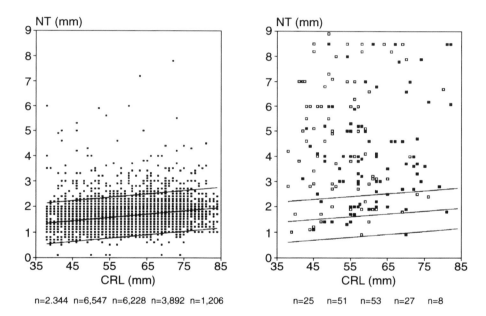

n=2.344 n=6,547 n=6,228 n=3,892 n=1,206   n=25   n=51   n=53   n=27   n=8

Figure 3.8 The multi-centre screening study. Fetal nuchal translucency (NT) in 20,217 chromosomally normal fetuses (left), in 86 fetuses with trisomy 21 (■ right) and in 78 fetuses with other chromosomal abnormalities (□ right) plotted on the reference range (median, 5th and 95th centiles) with crown–rump length (CRL).

For each measurement of translucency, the distance from the appropriate normal mean for crown–rump length (delta value) was determined. The distributions of delta nuchal translucency thickness in the chromosomally normal and trisomy 21 groups were examined (Figure 3.9).

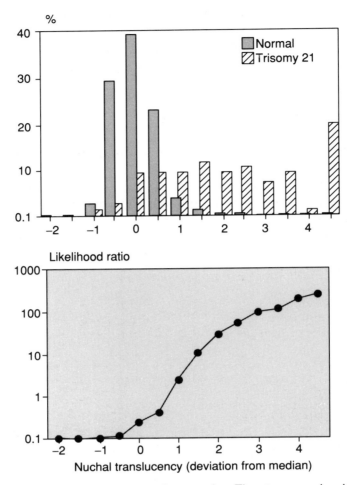

Figure 3.9 The multi-centre screening study. The top graph shows the distribution of fetal nuchal translucency expressed as deviation from the normal mean in 20,217 chromosomally normal fetuses (black bars) and 86 with trisomy 21 (hatched bars). The bottom graph shows likelihood ratios derived from the incidences in the two groups.

Likelihood ratios for trisomy 21 were determined by dividing the percentage of affected pregnancies with a given delta nuchal translucency by the percentage of normal pregnancies with the same delta nuchal translucency (Figure 3.9). Delta nuchal translucency was not associated with maternal age in either the chromosomally normal or the trisomy 21 group. Consequently, an estimate for an individual woman's risk based on her age and fetal nuchal translucency thickness can be calculated from her age-specific risk and likelihood ratio. Screening by this method of combining maternal age and fetal nuchal translucency thickness for a given crown–rump length identified 80% of the fetuses with trisomy 21 for a 5% screen positive rate.

Nuchal translucency and fetal heart rate

In a screening study of 8,980 pregnancies undergoing ultrasound examination for measurement of fetal nuchal translucency thickness at 10-14 weeks of gestation, the fetal heart rate was also measured (Hyett *et al* 1995a). In the normal group the fetal heart rate decreased with gestational age and in the fetuses with trisomy 21 the median fetal heart rate was significantly higher than in the normal pregnancies (mean difference, 5.5 bpm; t=4.2; p<0.0001) (Figure 3.10).

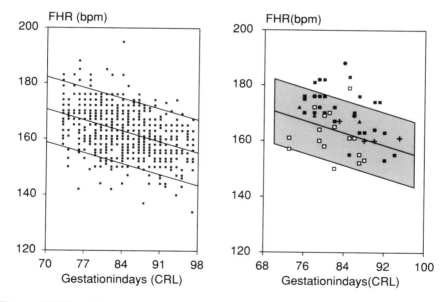

Figure 3.10 Fetal heart rate (FHR) plotted against gestation calculated from the crown–rump length in normal pregnancies (left). The lines indicate the normal mean, 5th and 95th centiles. On the right are the values from 43 pregnancies with trisomy 21 (■).

From the frequency distributions of fetal heart rate deviation from the appropriate normal mean for crown–rump length in the trisomy 21 and normal pregnancies, it was possible to derive likelihood ratios for trisomy 21 at different cut-off levels of heart rate (Figure 3.11).

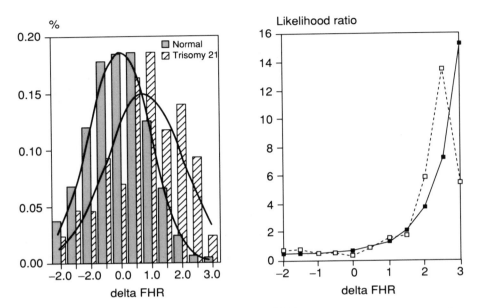

Figure 3.11 Distribution of fetal heart rate (FHR) measurements expressed as number of standard deviations from the normal mean for gestation in chromosomally normal fetuses and in fetuses with trisomy. On the right are the likelihood ratios for trisomy 21 in relation with delta FHR.

In both the trisomy 21 and the normal pregnancies there was no significant association between the nuchal translucency thickness and fetal heart rate. Therefore, fetal nuchal translucency and heart rate can be combined in calculating the risk for trisomies. It was estimated that in screening of the whole pregnant population by a combination of these two measurements as well as maternal age, 88% of trisomy 21 pregnancies can be detected for a screen positive rate of 5% (Hyett *et al* 1995a).

Nuchal translucency and maternal serum biochemistry

In trisomy 21 during the first trimester of pregnancy, the maternal serum concentration of free beta human chorionic gonadotrophin (free β-hCG) is higher and pregnancy associated plasma protein A (PAPP-A) is lower than in chromosomally normal pregnancies (Table 3.6; Figure 3.12).

Table 3.6 Maternal serum PAPP-A and free β-hCG in pregnancies with fetal trisomy 21 during the first trimester of pregnancy.

	Gestation	Trisomy 21	
		N	Median (MoM)
PAPP-A			
Wald *et al* 92	9-12 wks	19	0.23
Brambati *et al* 93	6-11 wks	14	0.30
Hurley *et al* 93	8-12 wks	7	0.33
Muller *et al* 93	9-14 wks	17	0.42
Bersinger *et al* 94	10-13 wks	29	0.53
Brizot *et al* 94	10-13 wks	45	0.50
Free β-hCG			
Ozturk *et al* 90	8-12 wks	9	1.60
Aitken *et al* 93	7-13 wks	14	2.00
Macri *et al* 90	10-13 wks	29	2.20
Macintosh *et al* 94	8-12 wks	14	2.10
Brizot *et al* 95	10-13 wks	41	2.00

Studies examining the relationship between maternal serum PAPP-A or free β-hCG concentrations and fetal nuchal translucency thickness have demonstrated no significant association between biochemistry and ultrasound findings in either the chromosomally normal or the trisomy 21 pregnancies (Figure 3.13; Brizot *et al* 1994, 1995). Therefore, maternal serum PAPP-A and free β-hCG and fetal nuchal translucency can be combined in calculating risks for fetal trisomies. It was estimated that such a method would identify about 90% of trisomy 21 pregnancies for a 5% screen positive rate.

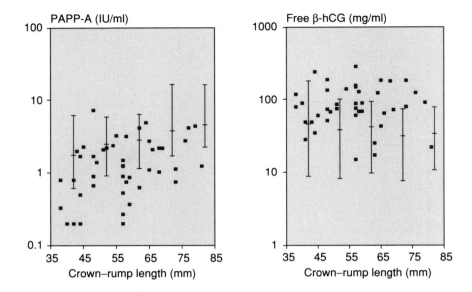

Figure 3.12 Maternal serum PAPP-A (left) and free β-hCG (right) in trisomy 21 pregnancies plotted on the normal range for fetal crown–rump length (mean, 95th and 5th centile). Adapted from Brizot *et al* 1994, 1995.

PATHOLOGICAL FINDINGS

Hyett *et al* (1995b) reported on the pathological examination of the fetal heart in 36 fetuses with trisomy 21 after suction termination of pregnancy at 12–15 weeks' gestation. The heart was identified and fixed by direct perfusion-inflation with paraformaldehyde, which was injected through the apex of each ventricle under microscopic control. Using a step-wise microdissection method and scanning electron microscopy, it was possible to examine the interventricular septum.

Perimembranous ventricular and atrioventricular septal defects (Figure 3.14) were detected in 56% of the cases; the incidence was approximately 10% in fetuses with nuchal translucency thickness of 3 mm and about 75% for the ones with translucency of 4 mm or more (Table 3.7). In two cases with translucency of 5 mm, the perimembranous ventricular septal defect was partly obliterated by the overlying septal leaflet of the tricuspid valve. The findings suggest that, although a septal defect may well be

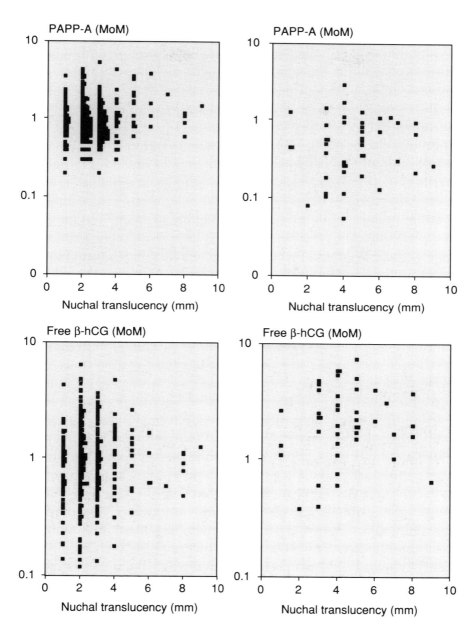

Figure 3.13 Relation of fetal nuchal translucency thickness and maternal serum PAPP-A (top) and free β-hCG (bottom) in the chromosomally normal groups (left) and those with trisomy 21 (right). The values are expressed as multiples of the median (MoM) for crown–rump length in the chromosomally normal group with fetal nuchal translucency thickness of less than 2.5 mm (adapted from Brizot *et al* 1994, 1995).

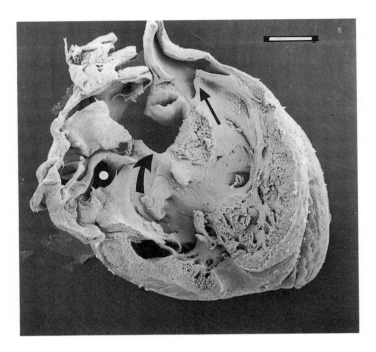

Figure 3.14 Photograph (magnification 29 times) demonstrating a ventricular septal defect (curved arrow) at 11 weeks of gestation. The pulmonary valve is bicuspid (straight arrow). The scale bar is 500 μm.

Table 3.7 Atrioventricular and perimembranous ventricular septal defects in fetuses with trisomy 21 in relation to the nuchal translucency thickness at diagnosis (from Hyett *et al* 1995).

Nuchal thickness	N	Septal defect		
		Any	Atrioventricular	Ventricular
3 mm	11	1	1	-
4 mm	7	5	2	3
5 mm	7	5	3	2
6 mm	1	1	1	-
7 mm	2	2	2	-
8 mm	3	3	2	1
9 mm	2	1	-	1
10 mm	1	1	1	-
12 mm	2	1	-	1
Total	**36**	**20**	**12**	**8**

implicated in the pathogenesis of nuchal translucency of 4 mm or more, it is unlikely to be responsible for a translucency of 3 mm.

The frequency of septal defects in trisomy 21 fetuses with increased nuchal translucency thickness at 10–14 weeks of gestation was twice as high as in live births with trisomy 21; echocardiographic studies in affected neonates reported atrioventricular or ventricular septal defects in about one third of cases (Hoe *et al* 1990, Tubman *et al* 1991).

It is possible that a high proportion of trisomy 21 fetuses with cardiac defects die *in utero*. Alternatively, there is spontaneous intrauterine closure of septal defects; postnatally, ventricular septal defects undergo spontaneous closure within 1 year in 45% of the cases (Moe *et al* 1987). Closure of perimembranous ventricular septal defects is thought to be due to adherence of the septal leaflet of the tricuspid valve to the margin of the defect (Anderson *et al* 1983), as observed in two of our cases.

A morphometric study of the great vessels in 34 trisomy 21 fetuses at 11-16 weeks of gestation has demonstrated that the diameter of the isthmus is narrower, whereas the aortic valve and ascending aorta are wider than in normal fetuses (Figure 3.15) (Hyett *et al* 1995c). Furthermore, there was a significant increase in the ratio of the diameter of the distal ductus arteriosus to that of the aortic isthmus (Figure 3.16).

Flow is related to vessel diameter and therefore widening of the ascending aorta together with narrowing of the aortic isthmus could lead to overperfusion of the tissues of the head and neck and may be responsible for the increased nuchal translucency thickness of trisomic fetuses. With advancing gestation, there is differential growth in the diameter of the great vessels, and the diameter of the aortic isthmus increases more rapidly than the diameters of the aortic valve and distal ductus (Hyett *et al* 1995d). Therefore, with increasing gestation, the haemodynamic consequences of narrowing of the isthmus may be overcome and this could offer an explanation for the gestational age-related spontaneous resolution of nuchal translucency.

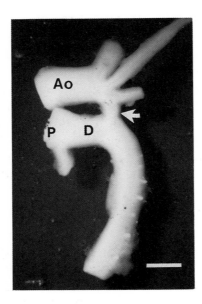

Figure 3.15 The aortic isthmus (arrow) is hypoplastic (white arrow) and the ductus arteriosus (D) is dilated in this trisomic fetus at 12 weeks of gestation. Ascending aorta (Ao). Pulmonary trunk (P). Scale bar: 3mm.

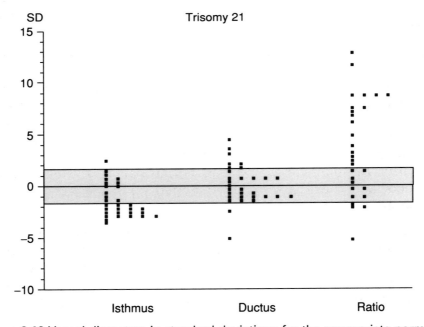

Figure 3.16 Vessel diameters in standard deviations for the appropriate normal mean for gestation at the aortic isthmus, distal ductus arteriosus and the ratio of ductus to isthmus in trisomy 21 fetuses. The shaded area represents the interval between the 10th and 90th centiles of the normal ranges.

EVOLUTION OF NUCHAL TRANSLUCENCY

Trisomy 21 fetuses

Screening for chromosomal defects in the first rather than the second trimester has the advantage of earlier prenatal diagnosis and consequently less traumatic termination of pregnancy for those couples that chose this option. A potential disadvantage is that earlier screening preferentially identifies those chromosomally abnormal pregnancies that are destined to miscarry. Snijders *et al* (1994) compared the prevalence of trisomy 21 at 9–14 weeks with that in live births and estimated that approximately 53% of affected fetuses die *in utero* (see Chapter 2).

In a study of 108 fetuses with trisomy 21 diagnosed in the first trimester because of increased nuchal translucency thickness, in five cases the parents chose to continue with the pregnancy whereas in 103 they had termination; trisomy 21 was also diagnosed in one of the fetuses in a twin pregnancy where the parents elected to avoid invasive prenatal diagnosis or selective fetocide (Pandya *et al* 1995e). The maternal age, ultrasound findings and outcome of the six trisomy 21 fetuses are shown in Table 3.8.

In five of the six fetuses the nuchal translucency resolved and at the second trimester scan the nuchal fold thickness was normal (less than 7 mm). At the second trimester scan, one fetus had nuchal oedema, three had septal defects, two had echogenic bowel and one had mild hydronephrosis or pyelectasia. All six trisomy 21 babies were born alive and five are healthy. One had a major atrioventricular septal defect and died at the age of 6 months. Another two of the babies had small ventricular septal defects and these are being managed conservatively awaiting spontaneous closure.

These data suggest that increased nuchal translucency does not necessarily identify those trisomic fetuses that are destined to die *in utero*. However, the number of cases is too small to draw conclusions on the relation between the thickness of nuchal translucency and the relative risk of intrauterine death in trisomy 21.

Table 3.8 Maternal age (MA), gestational age (GA), ultrasound findings (NT=nuchal translucency thickness, NF=nuchal fold thickness, VSD=ventricular-septal defect) and outcome including sex, anomalies, gestation at delivery and birth weight in six trisomy 21 fetuses with increased nuchal translucency thickness. In case 5 the baby had a large atrio-ventricular septal defect and died at the age of 6 months (Pandya *et al* 1995e).

Case	MA	GA	Ultrasound findings	Outcome
1	22	13	NT 10 mm	Healthy male
		20	NF 6 mm	37 wks, 2458 g
2	40	11	NT 7 mm	Healthy male
		18	NF 4 mm	37 wks, 3260 g
3	26	11	NT 5 mm	Female, small VSD
		21	NF 5 mm, echogenic bowel, septal defect	39 wks, 3934 g
4	27	12	NT 5 mm	Male small VSD
		20	NF 5 mm, echogenic bowel, pyelectasia, septal defect	39 wks, 3771 g
5	41	12	NT 4 mm	Female, large VSD
		18	NF 4 mm, septal defect	32 wks, 1640 g
6	40	12	NT 8 mm	Healthy female
		20	NF 8 mm	36 wks, 1510 g

Chromosomally normal fetuses

Johnson *et al* (1993) examined 27 chromosomally normal fetuses with increased nuchal translucency (≥2 mm). In 24 cases the translucency resolved by 18 weeks and in all but one, where the baby had Noonan syndrome, the babies were healthy. In two cases the pregnancies were terminated because there was progressive hydrops and there was one intrauterine death associated with obstructive uropathy. In a subsequent study of 22 chromosomally normal fetuses (which included 17 of the above 27 cases), there were four terminations of pregnancy (three because of progressive hydrops and one because of amnion dysruption sequence), one intrauterine death (the fetus with obstructive uropathy above), one spontaneous abortion and 16 live births (Trauffer *et al* 1994). The 16 infants included 13 healthy ones, two with non-specific dysmorphic features and one with Noonan syndrome.

Shulman *et al* (1994) reported on 32 chromosomally normal fetuses with increased nuchal translucency (≥2.5 mm). In one case there were persistent hygromas that were successfully repaired at birth and in the other 31 cases the translucency resolved by 20 weeks and all babies were healthy at birth; follow-up examination at 12 months demonstrated normal growth and development in all infants.

Pandya *et al* (1994, 1995d) reported on the outcome of 565 chromosomally normal fetuses with nuchal translucency 3–9 mm (Table 3.9). Survival decreased with nuchal translucency thickness from 97% for 3 mm to 53% for $\geq$5 mm. In all babies that survived, the translucency resolved by 20 weeks of gestation. One of the survivors has Stickler syndrome but all others were apparently healthy.

Termination of pregnancy was carried out in 21 of the 551 cases with translucency of 3–6 mm, because fetal abnormalities were detected either at presentation (such as anencephaly or major exomphalos) or at follow-up scans (mainly cardiac defects). Termination of pregnancy was also performed in nine of the 14 cases with translucency of 7–9 mm because of the uncertain prognosis; a repeat scan 2 weeks after presentation demonstrated persistence or increase in the translucency and development of generalised oedema.

The incidence of structural defects, mainly cardiac, diaphragmatic, renal and abdominal wall, was approximately 4%, which is higher than would be expected in an unselected population. It is therefore necessary that detailed ultrasound scans are performed to diagnose such defects. In this study, all patients also had an infection screen because congenital infection is a recognised cause of fetal hydrops and may certainly account for the transient nature of translucency. In three cases the maternal blood IgM was positive for parvo B19 virus, Coxsackie B virus and toxoplasmosis, respectively. In all three cases healthy infants were delivered at term; the mother with toxoplasmosis was treated with spiramycin.

The incidences of spontaneous miscarriage or perinatal death for nuchal translucency of 3 mm and 4 mm were 2% and 4%, respectively. These rates are similar to the 2.3% rate of fetal loss

Table 3.9 Outcome of chromosomally normal fetuses with nuchal translucency thickness at least 3 mm. IUD=intrauterine death, NND=neonatal death.

NT	N	Alive	Perinatal		Termination of pregnancy	
			n	Death	n	Abnormalities
3 mm	459	97%	9	IUD at 13wks IUD at 15wks IUD at 16wks IUD at 17wks IUD at 27wks IUD at 30wks IUD at 35wks NND at 28wks NND at 40wks	6	Diaphragmatic hernia at 16wks Hydrops at 18wks Tricuspid atresia at 20wks Obstructive uropathy at 14wks Renal agenesis at 20wks Multicystic kidneys at 20wks Ventriculomegaly at 22wks
4 mm	55	91%	2	IUD at 16wks IUD at 20wks	3	Exomphalos at 12wks Exomphalos at 13wks Hypoplastic left heart at 19wks
5 mm	24	63%*	3	IUD at 15wks IUD at 16wks NND at 38wks**	6	Hypoplastic left heart at 16wks Tricuspid atresia at 24wks Holoprosencephaly at 20wks Exomphalos at 13wks Gonadal dysgenesis at 23wks Hydrops at 13wks
6 mm	13	62%	-		5	Exomphalos at 13wks Anencephaly, exomphalos at 12wks Amnion dysruption sequence at 16wks Arthrogryposis at 16wks Hydrops at 20wks
7 mm	3	33%	1	NND at 35wks***	1	Hydrops at 12wks
8 mm	5	60%	-		2	Hydrops and talipes at 15wks Hydrops at 17wks
9 mm	6	-	-		6	Hydrops at 13wks Hydrops at 14wks Hydrops at 14wks Hydrops at 15wks Hydrops and septal defect at 16wks Hydrops at 20wks
Total	565	92%	15		29	

* One case where Stickler syndrome diagnosed postnatally, ** Diaphragmatic hernia diagnosed at 20 weeks, *** Charge syndrome diagnosed postnatally.

observed in a group of fetuses with normal nuchal translucency thickness undergoing chorion villus sampling (Nicolaides *et al* 1994a). In contrast, for fetal translucency of ≥ 5 mm the rate of fetal loss was increased (13%) and presumably this would have been even higher had termination not been performed for those cases that developed hydrops.

NUCHAL TRANSLUCENCY IN MULTIPLE PREGNANCIES

Screening for chromosomal defects by measurement of nuchal translucency thickness is particularly useful in multiple pregnancies because the alternative method of screening, by maternal serum biochemistry, is not applicable to such pregnancies.

Table 3.10 Maternal age (MA), method of conception, gestational age (GA) at presentation, fetal crown–rump length (CRL), nuchal translucency thickness (NT), fetal karyotype and outcome of the eight twin pregnancies.

Case	MA (yrs)	GA (wks)	CRL (mm)	NT (mm)	Karyotype	Outcome
1	35	13	82	2	47,XY+21	Termination
			78	8	47,XY+21	Termination
2	37	13	81	8	47,XY+21	Termination
			65	3	47,XX+18	Termination
3	43	12	38	7	47,XY+18	Embryo reduction
			49	2	46,XY	Termination
4	31	12	56	8	47,XX+21	Embryo reduction
			59	2	46,XY	Live birth 39 wk
5	35	11	54	4	47,XX+21	Embryo reduction
			57	2	46,XY	Live birth 39 wk
6	36	13	69	5	47,XX+21	Embryo reduction
			75	2	46,XY	Live birth 38 wk
7	21	12	69	5	47,XY+21	Embryo reduction
			65	2	46,XY	Live birth 40 wk
8	38	13	72	4	47,XY+21	Embryo reduction
			79	3	46,XY	Continuing

There is an additional advantage to first trimester scanning and measurement of nuchal translucency thickness in twin pregnancies: when one of the fetuses is found to have a chromosomal abnormality and the other is normal, the parents may choose to have selective termination of pregnancy. In such cases, the presence of a sonographically detectable marker ensures the correct identification of the abnormal twin. Furthermore, a recent multicentre study has demonstrated that embryo reduction before 16 weeks' gestation is associated with a much lower risk of miscarriage (5.4%) than selective termination after 16 weeks (14.4%; Evans *et al* 1994).

Therefore, in twin pregnancies complicated by the presence of a chromosomal abnormality in one of the fetuses, measurement of nuchal translucency thickness can help identify the affected twin and provide the option for selective fetocide in the first trimester.

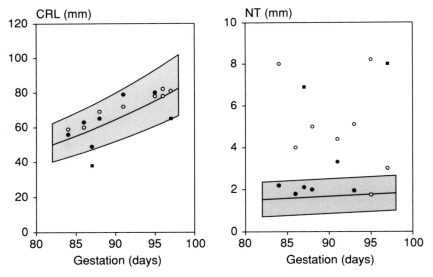

Figure 3.17 Crown–rump length (CRL) and nuchal translucency thickness (NT) of chromosomally normal fetuses (●) and in fetuses with trisomy 21 (o) and trisomy 18 (■) in twin pregnancies plotted on the appropriate reference range with gestation for singleton pregnancies (mean, 5th and 95th centile).

Pandya *et al* (1995c) examined the crown–rump length and nuchal translucency thickness of each fetus in eight twin pregnancies where karyotyping at 10–14 weeks of gestation demonstrated that at least one of the fetuses was chromosomally abnormal (Table 3.10). Eight fetuses had trisomy 21 and two had trisomy 18. The nuchal translucency thickness was more than 2.5 mm in nine (90%) of the trisomic fetuses and in one of the chromosomally normal ones (Figure 3.17). The crown–rump length was within the normal range for singleton pregnancies in 15 of the 16 fetuses. In one fetus with trisomy 18 the crown–rump length was below the 5th centile.

REFERENCES

Aitken DA, McCaw G, Crossley JA, Berry C, Connor JM, Spencer K, Macri JN. First-trimester biochemical screening for fetal chromosome abnormalities and neural tube defects. Prenat Diagn 1993; 13: 681-9.

Anderson RH, Lenox CC, Zubherbuhler JR. Mechanisms of closure of perimembranous ventricular septal defect. Am J Cardiol 1983; 52: 341-5.

Bergsio P, Denman III DW, Hoffman J, Meirik O. Duration of human singleton pregnancy. Acta Obstet Gynecol Scand 1990; 69: 197-207.

Bersinger NA, Brizot ML, Johnson A, Snijders RJM, Abbott J, Schneider H, Nicolaides KH. First trimester maternal serum pregnancy-associated plasma protein A and pregnancy-specific ß1-glycoprotein in fetal trisomies. Br J Obstet Gynaecol 1994; 101: 970-4.

Brambati B, Macintosh MCM, Teisner B, Maguiness S, Shrimanker K, Lanzani A, Bonacchi I, Tului L, Chard T, Grudzinskas TJ. Low maternal serum level of pregnancy associated plasma protein (PAPP-A) in the first trimester in association with abnormal fetal karyotype. Br J Obstet Gynaecol 1993; 100: 324-6.

Brambati B, Cislaghi C, Tului L, Alberti E, Amidani M, Colombo U, Zuliani G. First-trimester Down's syndrome screening using nuchal translucency: a prospective study. Ultrasound Obstet Gynecol 1995; 5: 9-14.

Brizot ML, Snijders RJM, Bersinger NA, Kuhn P, Nicolaides KH. Maternal serum pregnancy associated placental protein A and fetal nuchal translucency thickness for the prediction of fetal trisomies in early pregnancy. Obstet Gynecol 1994; 84: 918-22.

Brizot ML, Snijders RJM, Butler J, Bersinger NA, Nicolaides KH. Maternal serum hCG and fetal nuchal translucency thickness for the prediction of fetal trisomies in the first trimester of pregnancy. Br J Obstet Gynaecol 1995;102:127-32.

Bronshtein M, Rottem S, Yoffe N, Blumenfeld Z. First trimester and early second trimester diagnosis of nuchal cystic hygroma by transvaginal sono-graphy: Diverse prognosis of the septated from the non septated lesion. Am J Obstet Gynecol 1989; 161: 78-82.

Campbell S, Warsof SL, Little D, Cooper DJ. Routine ultrasound screening for the prediction of gestational age. Obstet Gynecol 1985; 65: 613-20.

Cohen MM, Schwartz S, Schwartz MF, Blitzer MG, Raffel LJ, Mullins Keene CL, Sun CC, Blakemore KJ. Antenatal detection of cystic hygroma. Obstet Gynecol Surv 1989; 44: 481-90.

Comas C, Martinez JM, Ojuel J, Casals E, Puerto B, Borrell A, Fortuny A. First-trimester nuchal edema as a marker of aneuploidy. Ultrasound Obstet Gynecol 1995; 5: 26-9.

Cullen MT, Gabrielli S, Green JJ, Rizzo N, Mahoney MJ, Salafia C, Bovicelli L, Hobbins JC. Diagnosis and significance of cystic hygroma in the first trimester. Prenat Diagn 1990; 10: 643-51.

Dallapiccola B, Zelante L, Perla G, Villani G. Prenatal diagnosis of recurrence of cystic hygroma with normal chromosomes. Prenat Diagn 1984; 4: 383-6.

Drugan A, Johnson MP, Isada NB, *et al.* The smaller than expected first-trimester fetus is at increased risk for chromosome anomalies. Am J Obstet Gynecol 1992; 167: 1525-8.

Evans MI, Goldberg JD, Dommergues M, Wapner RJ, Lynch L, Dock BS, Horenstein J, Golbus MS, Rodeck CH, Dumez Y, Holzgreve W, Timor-Tritsch T, Johnson MP, Isada NB, Monteagudo A, Berkowitz RL. Efficacy of second-trimester selective termination for fetal abnormalities: International collaborative experience among the world's largest centers. Am J Obstet Gynecol 1994; 171: 90-4.

Geirsson RT. Ultrasound instead of last menstrual period as the basis of gestational age assignment. Ultrasound Obstet Gynecol 1991; 1: 212-19.

Gustavii B, Edvall H. First-trimester diagnosis of cystic nuchal hygroma. Acta Obstet Gynecol Scand 1984; 63: 377-8.

Hewitt B. Nuchal translucency in the first trimester. Aust NZ J Obstet Gynaecol 1993; 33: 389-91.

Hill LM, Macpherson T, Rivello D, Peterson C. The spontaneous resolution of cystic hygromas and early fetal growth delay in fetuses with trisomy 18. Prenat Diagn 1991; 11: 673-7.

Hoe TS, Chan KC, Boo NY. Cardiovascular malformations in Malaysian neonates with Down's Syndrome. Singapore Med J 1990; 31: 474-6.

Hurley PA, Ward RHT, Teisner B, Iles RK, Lucas M, Grudzinkas JG. Serum PAPP-A measurements in first-trimester screening for Down syndrome. Prenat Diagn 1993; 13: 903-8.

Hyett JA, Noble PL, Snijders RJM, Montenegro N, Nicolaides KH. Fetal heart rate and trisomy 21 at 10–14 weeks of gestation. Ultrasound Obstet Gynecol 1995a (in press).

Hyett JA, Moscoso G, Nicolaides KH. First trimester nuchal translucency and cardiac septal defects in fetuses with trisomy 21. Am J Obstet Gynecol 1995b (in press).

Hyett JA, Moscoso G, Nicolaides KH. Increased nuchal translucency in trisomy 21 fetuses: Relation to narrowing of the aortic isthmus. Hum Reprod 1995c (in press).

Hyett JA, Moscoso G, Nicolaides KH. Morphometric analysis of the great vessels in early fetal life. Hum Reprod 1995d (in press).

Johnson MP, Johnson A, Holzgreve W, Isada NB, Wapner RJ, Treadwell MC, Heeger S, Evans M. First-trimester simple hygroma: Cause and outcome. Am J Obstet Gynecol 1993; 168: 156-61.

Kuhn P, Brizot M, Pandya PP, Snijders RJ, Nicolaides KH. Crown-rump length in chromosomally abnormal fetuses at 10 to 13 weeks' gestation. Am J Obstet Gynecol 1995;172:32–5.

Lynch L, Berkowitz RL. First trimester growth delay in trisomy 18. Am J Perinatol 1989; 6: 237-9.

Macintosh MC, Iles R, Teisner B, Sharma V, Chard T, Grudzinskas JG. Maternal serum human chorionic gonadotrophin and pregnancy associated plasma protein A, markers for fetal Down syndrome at 8-14 weeks. Prenat Diagn 1994; 14: 203-8.

MacLeod AM, McHugo JM. Prenatal diagnosis of nuchal cystic hygroma. Br J Radiol 1991; 64: 802-7.

Macri JN, Kasturi RV, Krantz DA, Cook EJ, Moore ND, Young JA, Romero K, Larsen JW. Maternal serum Down syndrome screening: free beta protein is a more effective marker than human chorionic gonadotrophin. Am J Obstet Gynecol 1990; 163: 1248-53.

Moe DG, Guntheroth WG. Spontaneous closure of uncomplicated ventricular septal defect. Am J Cardiol 1987; 60: 674-8.

Muller F, Cuckle H, Teisner B, Grudzinskas JG. Serum PAPP-A levels are depressed in women with fetal Down syndrome in early pregnancy. Prenat Diagn 1993; 13: 633-6.

Nadel A, Bromley B, Benacerraf BR. Nuchal thickening or cystic hygromas in first- and early second-trimester fetuses: prognosis and outcome. Obstet Gynecol 1993; 82: 43-8.

Nicolaides KH, Azar G, Byrne D, Mansur C, Marks K. Fetal nuchal translucency: ultrasound screening for chromosomal defects in first trimester of pregnancy. Br Med J 1992; 304: 867-9.

Nicolaides KH, Brizot ML, Patel F, Snijders RJM. Comparative study of chorion villus sampling and amniocentesis for fetal karyotyping at 10-13 weeks gestation. Lancet 1994a; 344: 435-9.

Nicolaides KH, Brizot ML, Snijders RJM. Fetal nuchal translucency: ultrasound screening for fetal trisomy in the first trimester of pregnancy. Br J Obstet Gynaecol 1994b; 101: 782-6.

Ozturk M, Milunsky A, Brambati B, Sachs ES, Miller S, *et al* Abnormal maternal serum levels of human chorionic gonadotropin free subunits in trisomy 18. Am J Med Genet 1990; 36: 480-3.

Pandya PP, Brizot ML, Kuhn P, Snijders RJM, Nicolaides KH. First trimester fetal nuchal translucency thickness and risk for trisomies. Obstet Gynecol 1994; 84: 420-3.

Pandya PP, Altman D, Brizot ML, Pettersen H, Nicolaides KH. Repeatability of measurement of fetal nuchal translucency thickness. Ultrasound Obstet. Gynecol 1995a; 5: 337–40.

Pandya PP, Goldberg H, Walton B, Riddle A, Shelley S, Snijders RJM, Nicolaides KH. The implementation of first trimester scanning at 10-13 weeks' gestation and the measurement of fetal nuchal translucency thickness in two maternity units. Ultrasound Obstet Gynecol 1995b; 5: 20-5.

Pandya PP, Hilbert F, Snijders RJM, Nicolaides KH. Nuchal translucency thickness and crown-rump length in twin pregnancies with chromosomally abnormal fetuses. J Ultrasound Med 1995c (in press).

Pandya PP, Kondylios A, Hilbert L, Snijders RJM, Nicolaides KH. Chromosomal defects and outcome in 1,015 fetuses with increased nuchal translucency. Ultrasound Obstet Gynecol 1995d; 5: 15-19.

Pandya PP, Snijders RJM, Johnson S, Nicolaides KH. Natural history of trisomy 21 fetuses with fetal nuchal translucency. Ultrasound Obstet Gynecol 1995e (in press).

Pons JC, Diallo AA, Eydoux P, Rais S, Doumerc S, Frydman R, Papiernik E. Chorionic villus sampling after first trimester diagnosis of fetal cystic hygroma colli. Eur J Obstet Gynecol Reprod Biol 1989; 33: 141-6.

Reuss A, Pijpers L, Schampers PTFM, Wladimiroff JW, Sachs ES. The importance of chorionic villus sampling after first trimester diagnosis of cystic hygroma. Prenat Diagn 1987a; 7: 299-301.

Reuss A, Pijpers L, van Swaaij E, Jahoda MGJ, Wladimiroff JW. First-trimester diagnosis of recurrence of cystic hygroma using a transvaginal ultrasound transducer. Case report. Eur J Obstet Gynecol Reprod Biol 1987b; 26: 271-3.

Rottem S, Bronshtein M, Thaler I, Brandes JM. First trimester transvaginal sonographic diagnosis of fetal anomalies. Lancet 1989; 1: 444-5.

Savoldelli G, Binkert F, Achermann J, Schmid W. Ultrasound screening for chromosomal anomalies in the first trimester of pregnancy. Prenat Diagn 1993; 13: 513-18.

Schulte-Vallentin M, Schindler H. Non-echogenic nuchal oedema as a marker in trisomy 21 screening. Lancet 1992; 339: 1053.

Sepulveda WH, Ciuffardi I. Early sonographic diagnosis of fetal cystic hygromata colli. J Perinat Med 1992; 20: 149-52.

Shulman LP, Emerson D, Felker R, Phillips O, Simpson J, Elias S. High frequency of cytogenetic abnormalities with cystic hygroma diagnosed in the first trimester. Obstet Gynecol 1992; 80: 80-2.

Shulman LP, Emerson DS, Grevengood C, Felker RE, Gross SJ, Phillips OP, Elias S. Clinical course and outcome of fetuses with isolated cystic nuchal lesions and normal karyotypes detected in the first trimester. Am J Obstet Gynecol 1994; 171: 1278-81.

Snijders RJM, Holzgreve W, Cuckle H, Nicolaides KH. Maternal age specific risk for trisomies at 9-14 weeks gestation. Prenat Diagn 1994; 14: 543-52.

Suchet IB, van der Westhuizen NG, Labatte MF. Fetal cystic hygromas: further insights into their natural history. Can Assoc Radiol J 1992; 6: 420-4.

Szabo J, Gellen J. Nuchal fluid accumulation in trisomy-21 detected by vaginosonography in first trimester. Lancet 1990; 336: 1133.

Trauffer ML, Anderson CE, Johnson A, Heeger S, Morgan P, Wapner RJ. The natural history of euploid pregnancies with first-trimester cystic hygromas. Am J Obstet Gynecol 1994; 170: 1279-84.

Tubman TRJ, Shields MD, Craig BG, Mulholland HC, Nevin NC. Congenital heart disease in Down's Syndrome: Two year prospective early screening study. Br Med J 1991; 302: 1425-7.

Ville Y, Lalondrelle C, Doumerc S, Daffos F, Frydman R, Oury JF, Dumez Y. First-trimester diagnosis of nuchal anomalies: significance and fetal outcome. Ultrasound Obstet Gynecol 1992; 2: 314-16.

Wald N, Stone R, Cuckle HS, Grudzinskas JG, Barkai G, Brambati B, Teisner B, Fuhrmann W. First trimester concentrations of pregnancy associated plasma protein A and placental protein 14 in Down's syndrome. Br Med J 1992; 305: 28.

Wald NJ, Smith D, Kennard A, Palomaki GE, Salonen R, Holzgreve W, Pejtsik B, Coombes EJ, Macini G, MacRae AR, Wyatt P, Roberson J. Biparietal diameter and crown-rump length in fetuses with Down's syndrome: implications for antenatal serum screening for Down's syndrome. Br J Obstet Gynaecol 1993; 100: 430-5.

Wilson RD, Venir N, Faquharson DF. Fetal nuchal fluid – physiological or pathological? – in pregnancies less than 17 menstrual weeks. Prenat Diagn 1992; 12: 755-63.

van Zalen-Sprock MM, van Vugt JMG, van Geijn HP. First-trimester diagnosis of cystic hygroma - course and outcome. Am J Obstet Gynecol 1992; 167: 94-8.

Diagnostic techniques

AMNIOCENTESIS
>Fetal loss
>Early amniocentesis

CHORIONIC VILLUS SAMPLING
>Fetal loss
>Limb reduction defects and oromandibular hypoplasia
>Late chorionic villus sampling

CORDOCENTESIS
>Fetal loss

EXPERIMENTAL TECHNIQUES
>Coelocentesis
>Transcervical flushing
>Detection of fetal cells in the maternal circulation

AMNIOCENTESIS

The feasibility of culture and karyotyping amniotic fluid cells was first demonstrated by Steele and Breg in 1966 and trisomy 21 was first detected prenatally by Valenti *et al* in 1968.

Early attempts at genetic amniocentesis were made transvaginally, but subsequently the transabdominal approach was adopted. In the 1960s amniocentesis was performed 'blindly'. In the 1970s and early 1980s ultrasound, initially static and subsequently real-time, was used to identify a placenta-free area for entry into a pocket of amniotic fluid. The position of this was marked on the maternal abdomen and after a variable length of time, in some studies up to 2 days, the operator would 'blindly' insert the needle. It is therefore not surprising that early reports on the use of ultrasound produced conflicting conclusions with some suggesting that it was actually detrimental (Karp *et al* 1977). Amniocentesis is now performed with continuous ultrasound guidance.

Fetal loss

Ager and Oliver (1986) reported a critical appraisal of all the studies on amniocentesis that were published during 1975–1985. There were 28 major national studies each involving at least 1,000 cases; the total fetal loss rate, including spontaneous abortion, intrauterine death and neonatal death, after amniocentesis ranged from 2.4% to 5.2%. In four of the 28 studies, there were matched controls that did not undergo amniocentesis; the total fetal loss rate ranged from 1.8% to 3.7%. Ager and Oliver (1986) estimated from these studies that the risk of fetal loss in the groups having amniocentesis was 0.2–2.1% higher than in the controls.

The only randomised, controlled trial was performed in Denmark (Tabor *et al* 1986). In this study, 4,606 low risk, healthy women, 25–34 years old, at 14–20 weeks of gestation, were randomly allocated to amniocentesis or ultrasound examination alone (Table 4.1). The total fetal loss rate in the patients having amniocentesis was 1% higher than in the controls. There were significant associations between spontaneous fetal loss and (i) puncture of the placenta, (ii) high maternal serum alpha-fetoprotein and (iii) discoloured amniotic fluid.

Table 4.1 Randomised study of amniocentesis at 16-20 weeks of gestation compared to controls having ultrasound examination only (Tabor *et al* 1986).

	Amniocentesis	Control
Spontaneous abortion	1.7%**	1%
Preterm delivery	4.1%	3.5%
Birthweight < 2,500 g	4.9%	4.5%
Talipes	0.8%	1.2%
RDS/pneumonia	1.8%*	0.8%

* $p<0.05$ **$p<0.01$

The Danish study also reported that amniocentesis was associated with an increased risk of respiratory distress syndrome and pneumonia in neonates (Tabor *et al* 1986). Although some studies have reported an increased incidence of talipes and dislocation of the hip in the amniocentesis group, this was not confirmed by the Danish study (Tabor *et al* 1986).

Early amniocentesis

In the late 1980s early amniocentesis (EA) was introduced and studies with complete pregnancy follow-up have reported that the procedure related rate of fetal loss was around 3–6%.

A recent prospective study has compared early amniocentesis (EA) with chorionic villus sampling (CVS) at 10–13 weeks of gestation in women with viable singleton pregnancies requesting first trimester fetal karyotyping because of advanced maternal age, parental anxiety or family history of chromosomal abnormality in the absence of parental chromosomal rearrangement (Nicolaides *et al* 1994). The patients were offered the option of EA or CVS, or randomisation into EA or CVS. EA was performed in 731 cases (493 by choice and 238 by randomisation) and CVS was performed in 570 cases (320 by choice and 250 by randomisation).

EA and CVS were performed (i) for the same indication, (ii) at the same gestational range, (iii) by the same group of operators, (iv) using essentially the same technique of transabdominal ultrasound-guided insertion of a 20-gauge needle, and (v) the samples were sent to the same laboratories. Successful sampling resulting in a non-mosaic cytogenetic result was the same for both EA and CVS (97.5%); furthermore, the intervals between sampling and obtaining results are similar for the two techniques. The main indication for repeat testing in the CVS group was mosaicism, whereas in the EA group it was failed culture; this failure was related to gestation at sampling: 5.3% at 10 weeks and 1.6% at 11–13 weeks (Table 4.2).

Table 4.2 Successful sampling and need for repeat testing in the groups that chose to have early amniocentesis or chorion villus sampling and in those that were randomised.

	Early amniocentesis n = 731	Chorionic villus sampling n = 570
Successful sampling	100%	99.3%
First insertion	98.2%	96.3%
Second insertion	1.8%	3.0%
Repeat testing needed	2.5%	2.5%
Maternal tissue	-	0.7%
Culture failure	2.3%	0.5%
Mosaic result	0.1%	1.2%

Spontaneous loss (intrauterine and neonatal death) after EA was approximately 3% higher than after CVS (Table 4.3). The gestation at delivery and birthweight of the infants after EA and CVS were similar and the frequencies of preterm delivery or low birthweight were not higher than would be expected in a normal population. In the EA group the incidence of talipes equinovarus (1.63%) was higher than in the CVS group (0.56%), but this difference was not significant.

Table 4.3 Pregnancy outcome in the groups that chose early amniocentesis or chorion villus sampling and in the group that was randomised.

	Total n = 1301	Amniocentesis n = 731	Chorionic villus sampling n = 570
Survival	93%	92.3%	94.0%
Total loss	6.8%	7.5%	6.0%
Spontaneous death	4.0%	5.3%	2.3%
Termination	2.8%	2.2%	3.7%
Chromosomal defect	2.4%	1.9%	3.0%
Normal karyotype	0.5%	0.3%	0.7%
No follow up	0.08%	0.1%	-

These data suggest that EA and CVS are equally effective in providing conclusive cytogenetic results but the 2–3% excess risk of fetal loss for EA over CVS means it is likely that CVS will become the established technique for prenatal karyotyping in the first trimester.

CHORIONIC VILLUS SAMPLING

Chorionic villus sampling (CVS) was first attempted in the late 1960s by hysteroscopy (Hahnemann *et al* 1968), but the technique was associated with low success in both sampling and karyotyping and was abandoned in favour of amniocentesis. In the 1970s the desire for early diagnosis led to the revival of CVS, which was initially carried out by aspiration via a cannula that was introduced 'blindly' into the uterus through the cervix (Tietung Group 1975), Subsequently, ultrasound guidance was used for the transcervical (Kazy *et al* 1982) or transabdominal (Smidt-Jensen & Hahnemann 1984) insertion of a variety of cannulae or biopsy forceps.

Fetal loss

Three randomized studies have examined the rate of fetal loss following first trimester CVS compared to that of amniocentesis at 16 weeks of gestation (MRC 1991, Lippman *et al* 1992, Smidt-Jensen *et al* 1992). In total more than 7,000 women were randomised in these studies and the results are presented in Table 4.4

Table 4.4 Total fetal loss rate in four randomised studies comparing first trimester chorion villus sampling with second trimester amniocentesis.

Study	N	CVS	Amnio
MRC, 1991	3201	14.0%	9.0%
Canadian study, 1992	2391	7.6%	7.1%
Danish study, 1992	2069	6.3%	7.0%
Finnish study, 1993	800	7.8%*	8.3%

*$p<0.01$

The results from centres experienced in both procedures demonstrated that fetal loss is no greater after first trimester CVS compared to second trimester amniocentesis. The most likely explanation for the increased loss after CVS in the MRC trial is the participation of many centres with little experience in this technique.

Limb reduction defects and oromandibular hypoplasia

In 1991 severe transverse limb abnormalities, micrognathia and microglossia were reported in five of 289 pregnancies that had CVS at less than 10 weeks of gestation (Firth *et al* 1991). Subsequently, a series of other reports confirmed the possible association between early CVS and fetal defects, and analysis of 75 such cases demonstrated a strong association between the severity of the defect and the gestation at CVS (Firth *et al* 1994). Thus, the median gestation at CVS was 8 weeks for those with amputation of the whole limb and 10 weeks for those with defects affecting the terminal phalanges (Figure 4.1). The background incidence of terminal transverse limb defects is about 1.8 per 10,000 live births (Froster-Iskenius & Baird 1989), and the incidence following early CVS is estimated at 1 in 200–1,000 cases.

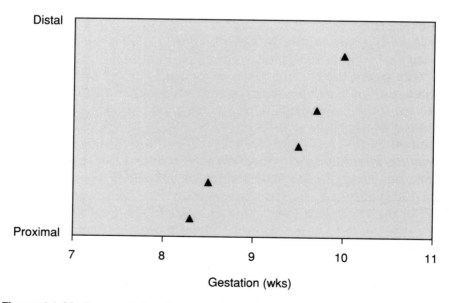

Figure 4.1 Median gestational age at chorionic villus sampling according to the level of reduction defect. Adapted from Firth *et al* (1994).

The types of defects are compatible with the pattern of limb development, which is essentially completed by the 10th week of gestation. Possible mechanisms by which early CVS may lead to limb defects include hypoperfusion, embolisation or release of vasoactive substances (Kuliev *et al* 1993, Rodeck 1993) and all these mechanisms are related to trauma. It is therefore imperative that CVS is performed only after 11 weeks by appropriately trained operators.

Late chorionic villus sampling

Although the main use of CVS is to obtain fetal tissue for early prenatal diagnosis, the same technique can also be used throughout pregnancy (Nicolaides *et al* 1986b). In a series of 225 cases of second and third trimester CVS, Holzgreve *et al* (1990) reported successful karyotyping in 99% of cases. More recently, a study of 551 women who had mid-trimester CVS reported adequate results for karyotyping in 99.6% of cases and the fetal loss rate after the procedure was only 0.4%, which may be lower than the loss rate following mid-trimester amniocentesis (Cameron *et al* 1994).

CORDOCENTESIS

Access to the fetal circulation was originally achieved by exposing the fetus at the time of hysterotomy (Freda and Adamsons 1964). Subsequently with the development of fibreoptics, fetoscopy was used to visualise and sample vessels on the chorionic plate (Hobbins and Mahoney 1974) and the umbilical cord (Rodeck and Campbell 1979). In the 1980s, ultrasound guidance made fetoscopy unnecessary; fetal blood can be obtained by ultrasound-guided puncture of an umbilical cord vessel (*cordocentesis*; Daffos *et al* 1983), intrahepatic umbilical vein (*hepatocentesis*; Bang *et al* 1982) or the fetal heart (*cardiocentesis*; Westgren *et al* 1988).

Cordocentesis can be performed by a single operator in an out-patient setting in the ultrasound department without need for maternal fasting, sedation, antibiotics and tocolytics or fetal paralysis (Nicolaides *et al* 1986a). In cases where the placenta is anterior or lateral, the needle is introduced transplacentally into the umbilical cord. When the placenta is posterior, the needle is introduced transamniotically and the cord punctured close to its placental insertion.

Fetal loss

The risk of fetal death after cordocentesis depends on the indication for sampling and the experience of the operator. Thus, Maxwell *et al* (1991), after excluding pregnancies that were terminated, noted that the fetal loss rates within 2 weeks of sampling were 1%, 7%, 14% and 25% in groups of structurally normal, structurally abnormal, growth retarded and hydropic fetuses, respectively.

In a series of 1169 cases (sampled for prenatal diagnosis of genetic disease, e.g. beta thalassaemia, or for karyotyping in cases of minor fetal malformations, e.g. hydronephrosis) there were 13 (1%) fetal losses within 2 weeks of the procedure; in addition there were 17 (1%) perinatal deaths at 4–20 weeks after cordocentesis (Nicolaides *et al* 1994).

Daffos *et al* (1985) in a series of 562 cases, sampled primarily for diagnosis of toxoplasmosis, reported seven fetal losses. Weiner *et al* (1991) reported no losses in 'salvageable' fetuses after cordocentesis in 594 cases. Boulot *et al* (1990) had ten fetal losses in 322 cases undergoing cordocentesis for a variety of indications.

EXPERIMENTAL TECHNIQUES

Coelocentesis

During the first trimester of pregnancy the amniotic sac is surrounded by the exocoelomic cavity which is a derivative of the extra-embryonic mesoderm. A study examining the feasibility of obtaining coelomic fluid by transvaginal insertion of a 20-gauge needle reported successful aspiration in nearly all cases at 6–10 weeks of gestation, in 40% of cases at 11 weeks and only 5% at 12 weeks (Jurkovic *et al* 1993).

Examination of the fluid demonstrated that, although cells from the exocoelomic cavity cannot be successfully cultured, embryonic genetic material can be analysed using fluorescent *in-situ* hybridisation (FISH) and polymerase chain reaction (PCR) techniques (Jurkovic *et al* 1993, Pandya *et al* 1994). However, diagnosis by FISH is restricted to chromosomal aneuploidies involving chromosomes X, Y, 13, 18 and 21, which may comprise between 66% and 88% of the chromosomal defects diagnosed by mid-trimester amniocentesis or first trimester chorionic villus sampling (Clark *et al* 1993; Snijders *et al* 1994).

The safety of coelocentesis is unknown and at present this technique remains experimental.

Transcervical flushing

In the early 1970s, studies examining the feasibility of isolating exfoliated placental cells in the cervical mucus using cotton swabs reported contradictory results. Shettles (1971) used a fluorescent dye test for detection of the Y chromosome and correctly diagnosed the fetal sex in 10 of 18 pregnancies investigated. However, using the same procedure, Bobrow and Lewis (1971) were unable to confirm these results, although Warren *et al* (1972) reported that the test was *'extremely easy to perform and accurate'.*

Subsequent studies have reported reasonable success in identifying placental cells by flushing mucus from the cervical canal or the lower uterine cavity (Griffith-Jones 1992, Morris 1992, Adinolfi *et al* 1993). Using monoclonal antibodies against placental cells it has been possible to isolate fetal cells from maternal contaminants by flow cytometry or magnetic beads. After purification, the cells could potentially be used for the prenatal diagnosis of a variety of inherited disorders.

Although the technique of obtaining these samples has been referred to as non-invasive, in reality it is not dissimilar to transcervical CVS because sampling success has been consistently achieved only when a cannula is introduced into the lower uterine cavity. The safety of this invasive test and the feasibility of producing reliable results remain to be established.

In a study of 20 pregnancies at 7–11 weeks of gestation, cervical lavage resulted in the recovery of trophoblastic cells from 50% of the cases (Bahado-Singh *et al* 1995). The technique has also been used for confirmation of trisomy 18 in a pregnancy where the diagnosis was originally made by CVS (Adinolfi *et al* 1993), and in the determination of rhesus type in fetuses from red cell isoimmunised pregnancies (Adinolfi *et al* 1995).

Detection of fetal cells in the maternal circulation

Fetal lymphocytes, nucleated erythrocytes and trophoblastic cells found in maternal blood can potentially be isolated for genetic diagnosis. However, the ratio of fetal to maternal cells in the maternal circulation is less than 1 in 5,000 (Ganshirt-Ahlert *et al* 1990) and at present there are no specific fetal cell surface markers.

Various techniques have been developed to separate fetal from maternal cells, including fluorescence activated cell sorting (Herzenberg *et al* 1979, Covone *et al* 1984, Bianchi *et al* 1990), density centrifugation (Goodfellow *et al* 1982) and magnetic cell sorting (Ganshirt-Ahlert *et al* 1992). Although these techniques result in enrichment of the proportion of fetal cells, the sample is unsuitable for cytogenetic analysis because it is still highly contaminated with maternal cells. The technique remains experimental and it is unlikely to replace invasive testing in the near future.

REFERENCES

Adinolfi M, Davies A, Sharif S, Soothill P, Rodeck CH. Detection of trisomy 18 and Y-derived sequences in fetal nucleated cells obtained by transcervical flushing. Lancet 1993;342:403-4.

Adinolfi M, Sherlock J, Kemp T, Carritt B, Soothill P, Kingdom J, Rodeck C. Prenatal detection of fetal Rh DNA sequences in transcervical samples. Lancet 1995;345:318-19.

Ager RP, Oliver RW. In: The risks of mid-trimester amniocentesis, being a comparative, analytical review of the major clinical studies. (Salford). 1986 197p.

Bahado-Singh RO, Kliman H, Feng TY, Hobbins J, Copel JA, Mahoney MJ. First trimester endocervical irrigation: feasibility of obtaining trophoblast cells for prenatal diagnosis. Obstet Gynecol 1995;85:461-4.

Bang J, Bock JE, Trolle D. Ultrasound-guided fetal intravenous transfusion for severe rhesus haemolytic disease. Br Med J 1982;284:373-4.

Bianchi DW, Flint AF, Pizzimenti MF, Knoll JHM, Latt SA. Isolation of fetal DNA from nucleated erythrocytes in maternal blood. Proc Natl Acad Sci USA 1990;87:3279-83.

Bobrow M, Lewis BV. Unreliability of fetal sexing using cervical material. Lancet 1971;ii:486.

Boulot P, Deschamps F, Lefort G, Sarda P, Mares P, Hedon B, Laffargue F, Viala JL. Pure fetal blood samples obtained by cordocentesis: technical aspects of 322 cases. Prenat Diagn 1990;10:93-100.

Cameron AD, Murphy KW, McNay MB, Mathers AM, Kingdom J, Aitken DA, Crossley J, Imrie S, Lowther G. Midtrimester chorionic villus sampling: an alternative approach? Am J Obstet Gynecol 1994;171:1035-7.

Canadian collaborative CVS-amniocentesis clinical trial group. Multicentre randomised clinical trial of chorion villus sampling and amniocentesis. Lancet 1989;i:1-6.

Clark BA, Kennedy K, Olson S. The need to reevaluate trisomy screening for advanced maternal age in prenatal diagnosis. Am J Obstet Gynecol 1993;168:812-16.

Covone AE, Mutton D, Johnson PM, Adinolfi M. Trophoblast cells in peripheral blood from pregnant women. Lancet 1984;2:841-3.

Daffos F, Capella Pavlovsky M, Forestier F. A new procedure for fetal blood sampling in utero: preliminary results of fifty-three cases. Am J Obstet Gynecol 1983;146:985-6.

Daffos F, Capella-Pavlovsky M, Forestier F. Fetal blood sampling during pregnancy with use of a needle guided by ultrasound: a study of 606 consecutive cases. Am J Obstet Gynecol 1985;153:655-60.

Firth HV, Boyd PA, Chamberlain P, MacKenzie IZ, Lindenbaum RH, Huson SM. Severe limb abnormalities after chorion villous sampling at 56-66 days' gestation. Lancet 1991;337:762-3.

Firth HV, Boyd PA, Chamberlain PF, MacKenzie IZ, Morriss-Kay GM, Huson SM. Analysis of limb reduction defects in babies exposed to chorion villus sampling. Lancet 1994;343:1069-71.

Freda VJ, Adamsons Jr. K. Exchange transfusions in utero. Am J Obstet Gynecol 1964;89:17-21.

Froster-Iskenius UG, Baird PA. Limb reduction defects in over one million consecutive livebirths. Teratology 1989;39:127-35.

Ganshirt-Ahlert D, Pohlschmidt M, Gal A, Miny P, Horst J, Holzgreve W. Ratio of fetal to maternal DNA is less than 1 in 5000 at different gestational ages in maternal blood. Clin Genet 1990;38:38-43.

Ganshirt-Ahlert D, Burschyk M, Garritsen HSP, Helmer L, Miny P, Horst J, Schneider HPG, Holzgreve W. Magnetic cell sorting and the transferrin receptor as potential means of prenatal diagnosis from maternal blood. Am J Obstet Gynecol 1992;166:1350-5.

Goodfellow CF, Taylor PV. Extraction and identification of trophoblast cells circulating in peripheral blood during pregnancy. Br J Obstet Gynaecol 1982;89:65-8.

Griffith-Jones MD, Miller D, Lilford RJ, Scott J. Detection of fetal DNA in trans-cervical swabs from first trimester pregnancies by gene amplification: a new route to prenatal diagnosis? Br J Obstet Gynaecol 1992;99:508-11.

Hahnemann N, Mohr J. Genetic diagnosis in the embryo by means of biopsy from extra embryonic membranes. Bull Eur Soc Hum Genet 1968;2:23 .

Herzenberg LA, Bianchi DW, Schroder J, Cann HM, Iverson GM. Fetal cells in the blood of pregnant women: detection and enrichment by fluorescence-activated cell sorting. Proc Natl Acad Sci USA 1979;76:1453-5.

Hobbins JC, Mahoney MJ. In utero diagnosis of hemoglobinopathies. Technic for obtaining fetal blood. N Engl J Med 1974;290:1065-7.

Holzgreve W, Miny P, Gerlach B. Benefits for rapid fetal karyotyping in the second and third trimester (late chorionic villus sampling) in high risk pregnancies. Am J Obstet Gynecol 1990;162:1188-92.

Jurkovic D, Jauniaux E, Campbell S, Pandya P, Cardy D, Nicolaides KH. Coelocentesis: a new technique for early prenatal diagnosis. Lancet 1993;341:1623-4.

Karp LE, Hayden PW. Fetal puncture during mid-trimester amniocentesis. Obstet Gynecol 1977;49:115.

Kazy Z, Rozovsky IS, Bakarev VA. Chorion biopsy in early pregnancy: a method of early prenatal diagnosis for inherited disorders. Prenat Diagn 1982;2:39.

Kuliev AM, Modell B, Jackson L, Simpson JL, Brambati B, Rhoads G, Froster U, Verlinsky Y, Smidt-Jensen S, Holzgreve W, Ginsberg N, Ammala P, Dumez Y. Risk evaluation of CVS. Prenat Diagn 1993;13:197-209.

Lippman A, Tomkins J, Shime J, Hamerton JL. Canadian multicentre randomized clinical trial of chorion villus sampling and amniocentesis. Prenat Diagn 1992;12:385-476.

Maxwell DJ, Johnson P, Hurley P. Fetal blood sampling and pregnancy loss in relation to indication. Br J Obstet Gynaecol 1991;98:892-7.

Morris N, Williamson R. Non-invasive first trimester antenatal diagnosis. Br J Obstet Gynaecol 1992;99:446-8.

MRC working party on the evaluation of chorion villus sampling. Medical Research Council European trial of chorion villus sampling. Lancet 1991;337:1491-9.

Nicolaides KH, Soothill PW, Rodeck CH, Campbell S. Ultrasound guided sampling of umbilical cord and placental blood to assess fetal wellbeing. Lancet 1986a;i:1065-7.

Nicolaides KH, Soothill PW, Rodeck CH. Why confine chorionic villus (placental) biopsy to the first trimester? Lancet 1986b;i:543-4.

Nicolaides KH, Brizot M, Patel F, Snijders R. Comparison of chorionic villus sampling and amniocentesis for fetal karyotyping at 10-13 weeks' gestation. Lancet 1994;344:435-9.

Pandya PP, Kuhn P, Brizot M, Cardy DL, Nicolaides KH. Rapid detection of chromosome aneuploidies in fetal blood and chorionic villi by fluorescence in situ hybridisation. Br J Obstet Gynaecol 1994;101:493-7.

Rodeck CH, Campbell S. Umbilical cord insertion as source of pure fetal blood for prenatal diagnosis. Lancet 1979;i:1244-5.

Rodeck CH. Fetal development after chorionic villus sampling. Lancet 1993;341:468-9.

Shettles LB. Use of the Y chromosome in prenatal sex determination. Nature 1971;230:52.

Smidt-Jensen S, Hahnemann N. Transabdominal fine needle biopsy from chorionic villi in first trimester. Prenat Diagn 1984;4:163.

Smidt-Jensen S, Permin M, Philip J, Lundsteen C, Zachary JM, Fowler SE, Gruning K. Randomised comparison of amniocentesis and transabdominal and transcervical chorionic villus sampling. Lancet 1992;340:1238-44.

Snijders RJ, Holzgreve W, Cuckle H, Nicolaides KH. Maternal age-specific risks for trisomies at 9-14 weeks' gestation. Prenat Diagn 1994;14:543-52.

Steele MW, Breg WR. Chromosome analysis of human amniotic-fluid cells. Lancet 1966;i:383-5.

Tabor A, Philip J, Madsen M, Bang J, Obel EB, Norgaard-Pedersen B. Randomised controlled trial of genetic amniocentesis in 4,606 low-risk women. Lancet 1986;i:1287-93.

Tietung Group, Anshan, China. Fetal sex prediction by sex chromatin of chorionic villi cells during early pregnancy. China Med J 1975;1:117.

Valenti C, Schutta EJ, Kehaty T. Prenatal diagnosis of Down's syndrome. Lancet 1968;ii:220.

Warren R, Sanchez L, Hammond D, McLeod A. Prenatal sex determination from exfoliated cells found in cervical mucus. Am J Hum Genet 1972;24:22a.

Weiner CP, Wenstrom KD, Sipes SL, Williamson RA. Risk factors for cordocentesis and fetal intravascular transfusion. Am J Obstet Gynecol 1991;165:1020-5.

Westgren M, Selbing A, Stangenberg M. Fetal intracardiac transfusions in patients with severe rhesus isoimmunisation. Br Med J Clin Res 1988;296:885-6.

Appendix 1:
Fetal biometry at
14–40 weeks of gestation

The normal ranges for fetal biometry presented in this section were established from cross-sectional data on 1,040 singleton pregnancies at 14–40 weeks gestation (Snijders & Nicolaides 1994). The patients fulfilled the following criteria: (i) known last menstrual period with a cycle length of 26–30 days, (ii) no fetal abnormalities and no pregnancy complications, (iii) live birth at term, (iv) birthweight above the 3rd and below the 97th centile for gestation (Yudkin et al 1987). For each 7-day interval from 14 to 40 weeks, 40 patients were included.

Measurements of biparietal diameter (BPD), occipito-frontal diameter (OFD), anterior and posterior cerebral ventricle diameter (Va and Vp), and hemisphere (H) were obtained from a transverse axial plane of the fetal head showing a central midline echo broken in the anterior third by the cavum septii pellucidi and demonstrating the anterior and posterior horns of the lateral ventricles. BPD and OFD were measured from the outer borders of the skull and head circumference (HC) was calculated [3.14 x (BPD+OFD)/2]. Va was the distance between the lateral wall of the anterior horn to the midline and Vp was the distance between the medial and lateral walls of the posterior horn. The hemisphere was measured from the midline to the inner border of the skull. Transverse cerebellar diameter (TCD) and cisterna magna diameter (CM) were measured in the suboccipito-bregmatic plane of the head. The femur length (FL) was measured from the greater trochanter to the lateral condyle. For abdominal circumference (AC), a transverse section of the fetal abdomen was taken at the level of the stomach and the bifurcation of the main portal vein into its right and left branches. The anteroposterior (AD1) and transverse (AD2) diameters were measured and AC was calculated [3.14 x (AD1+AD2)/2]. The following ratios were calculated, HC/AC, BPD/FL, HC/FL, AC/FL, TCD/HC, TCD/AC, BPD/OFD, Va/H and Vp/H.

For each of the measurements and their ratios, regression analysis was applied examining linear, quadratic and cubic models for the association with gestational age (in days). For those measurements where the standard deviation increased or decreased with gestation, logarithmic or square root transformation was applied to stabilise variance. If the quadratic or cubic terms did not improve the original linear model (an independent correlation with $p < 0.05$ and improvement of the correlation coefficient), the linear model was chosen as the best fit. Where the quadratic or cubic components did improve the model, they were included in the equation for the regression line. Equations for regression lines on transformed data were used to calculate the mean and residual SD in transformed units. To produce the reference ranges in the original units, the mean and limits of the calculated reference range in transformed units were subjected to anti-logarithmic or power transformation as appropriate.

Snijders RJ, Nicolaides KH. Fetal biometry at 14-40 weeks of gestation. Ultrasound Obstet Gynecol 1994;4:34-48.

Table 1 Abdominal circumference (mm).

Gestation	5th	median	95th
14+0 - 14+6	80	90	102
15+0 - 15+6	88	99	112
16+0 - 16+6	96	108	122
17+0 - 17+6	105	118	133
18+0 - 18+6	114	128	144
19+0 - 19+6	123	139	156
20+0 - 20+6	133	149	168
21+0 - 21+6	143	161	181
22+0 - 22+6	153	172	193
23+0 - 23+6	163	183	206
24+0 - 24+6	174	195	219
25+0 - 25+6	184	207	233
26+0 - 26+6	195	219	246
27+0 - 27+6	205	231	259
28+0 - 28+6	216	243	272
29+0 - 29+6	226	254	285
30+0 - 30+6	237	266	298
31+0 - 31+6	246	277	310
32+0 - 32+6	256	287	322
33+0 - 33+6	265	297	334
34+0 - 34+6	274	307	345
35+0 - 35+6	282	316	355
36+0 - 36+6	289	324	364
37+0 - 37+6	295	332	372
38+0 - 38+6	302	339	380
39+0 - 39+6	307	345	387

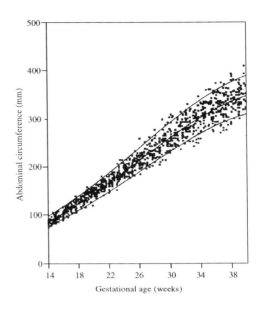

Table 2 Femur length (mm).

Gestation	5th	median	95th
14+0 - 14+6	14	17	19
15+0 - 15+6	17	19	22
16+0 - 16+6	19	22	25
17+0 - 17+6	21	24	28
18+0 - 18+6	24	27	30
19+0 - 19+6	26	30	33
20+0 - 20+6	29	32	36
21+0 - 21+6	32	35	39
22+0 - 22+6	34	38	42
23+0 - 23+6	37	41	45
24+0 - 24+6	39	43	47
25+0 - 25+6	42	46	50
26+0 - 26+6	44	48	53
27+0 - 27+6	47	51	55
28+0 - 28+6	49	53	58
29+0 - 29+6	51	56	60
30+0 - 30+6	53	58	63
31+0 - 31+6	55	60	65
32+0 - 32+6	57	62	67
33+0 - 33+6	59	64	69
34+0 - 34+6	61	66	71
35+0 - 35+6	63	68	73
36+0 - 36+6	64	69	74
37+0 - 37+6	66	71	76
38+0 - 38+6	67	72	77
39+0 - 39+6	68	73	78

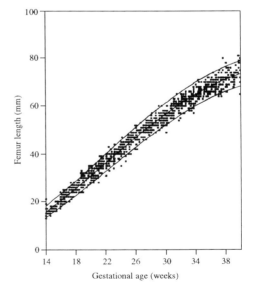

Table 3 Biparietal diameter (mm).

Gestation	5th	median	95th
14+0 - 14+6	28	31	34
15+0 - 15+6	31	34	37
16+0 - 16+6	34	37	40
17+0 - 17+6	36	40	43
18+0 - 18+6	39	43	47
19+0 - 19+6	42	46	50
20+0 - 20+6	45	49	54
21+0 - 21+6	48	52	57
22+0 - 22+6	51	56	61
23+0 - 23+6	54	59	64
24+0 - 24+6	57	62	68
25+0 - 25+6	60	66	71
26+0 - 26+6	63	69	75
27+0 - 27+6	66	72	78
28+0 - 28+6	69	75	81
29+0 - 29+6	72	78	85
30+0 - 30+6	74	81	88
31+0 - 31+6	77	83	90
32+0 - 32+6	79	86	93
33+0 - 33+6	81	88	96
34+0 - 34+6	83	90	98
35+0 - 35+6	85	92	100
36+0 - 36+6	86	94	102
37+0 - 37+6	87	95	103
38+0 - 38+6	88	96	104
39+0 - 39+6	89	97	105

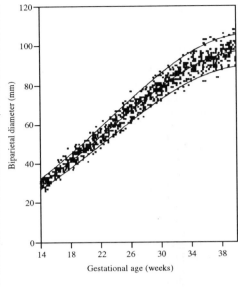

Table 4 Occipitofrontal diameter (mm).

Gestation	5th	median	95th
14+0 - 14+6	35	39	42
15+0 - 15+6	39	42	46
16+0 - 16+6	42	46	50
17+0 - 17+6	46	50	54
18+0 - 18+6	50	54	59
19+0 - 19+6	54	58	63
20+0 - 20+6	57	62	68
21+0 - 21+6	61	67	72
22+0 - 22+6	65	71	77
23+0 - 23+6	69	75	82
24+0 - 24+6	73	79	86
25+0 - 25+6	77	83	90
26+0 - 26+6	81	87	95
27+0 - 27+6	84	91	99
28+0 - 28+6	87	95	103
29+0 - 29+6	91	98	107
30+0 - 30+6	94	102	110
31+0 - 31+6	96	105	113
32+0 - 32+6	99	107	116
33+0 - 33+6	101	110	119
34+0 - 34+6	103	112	121
35+0 - 35+6	105	113	123
36+0 - 36+6	106	115	124
37+0 - 37+6	107	116	125
38+0 - 38+6	107	116	126
39+0 - 39+6	107	116	126

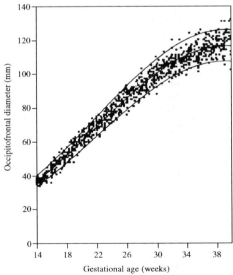

Table 5 Head circumference (mm).

Gestation	5th	median	95th
14+0 - 14+6	102	110	118
15+0 - 15+6	111	120	129
16+0 - 16+6	120	130	140
17+0 - 17+6	130	141	152
18+0 - 18+6	141	152	164
19+0 - 19+6	151	163	176
20+0 - 20+6	162	175	189
21+0 - 21+6	173	187	201
22+0 - 22+6	184	198	214
23+0 - 23+6	195	210	227
24+0 - 24+6	206	222	240
25+0 - 25+6	217	234	252
26+0 - 26+6	227	245	264
27+0 - 27+6	238	256	277
28+0 - 28+6	248	267	288
29+0 - 29+6	257	277	299
30+0 - 30+6	266	287	309
31+0 - 31+6	274	296	319
32+0 - 32+6	282	304	328
33+0 - 33+6	288	311	336
34+0 - 34+6	294	317	342
35+0 - 35+6	299	323	348
36+0 - 36+6	303	327	353
37+0 - 37+6	306	330	356
38+0 - 38+6	308	332	358
39+0 - 39+6	309	333	359

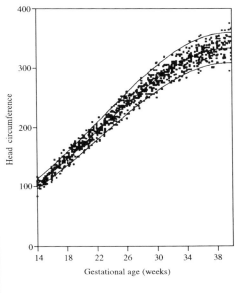

Table 6 Transverse cerebellar diameter (mm).

Gestation	5th	median	95th
14+0 - 14+6	12	14	15
15+0 - 15+6	13	15	17
16+0 - 16+6	14	16	18
17+0 - 17+6	15	17	19
18+0 - 18+6	16	18	21
19+0 - 19+6	17	20	22
20+0 - 20+6	19	21	24
21+0 - 21+6	20	22	25
22+0 - 22+6	21	24	27
23+0 - 23+6	22	25	28
24+0 - 24+6	24	26	30
25+0 - 25+6	25	28	31
26+0 - 26+6	26	29	33
27+0 - 27+6	27	31	34
28+0 - 28+6	29	32	36
29+0 - 29+6	30	33	37
30+0 - 30+6	31	35	39
31+0 - 31+6	32	36	40
32+0 - 32+6	34	37	42
33+0 - 33+6	35	39	43
34+0 - 34+6	36	40	44
35+0 - 35+6	37	41	46
36+0 - 36+6	38	42	47
37+0 - 37+6	39	43	48
38+0 - 38+6	40	44	49
39+0 - 39+6	41	45	51

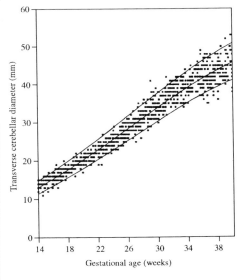

Page 175

Table 7 Cisterna magna diameter (mm).

Gestation	5th	median	95th
14+0 - 14+6	1.9	3.5	5.3
15+0 - 15+6	2.1	3.8	5.7
16+0 - 16+6	2.4	4.1	6.0
17+0 - 17+6	2.6	4.3	6.3
18+0 - 18+6	2.8	4.6	6.6
19+0 - 19+6	3.1	4.9	6.9
20+0 - 20+6	3.3	5.1	7.2
21+0 - 21+6	3.5	5.4	7.5
22+0 - 22+6	3.7	5.6	7.7
23+0 - 23+6	3.9	5.8	8.0
24+0 - 24+6	4.1	6.0	8.2
25+0 - 25+6	4.3	6.2	8.5
26+0 - 26+6	4.4	6.4	8.7
27+0 - 27+6	4.6	6.6	8.9
28+0 - 28+6	4.7	6.8	9.1
29+0 - 29+6	4.9	6.9	9.3
30+0 - 30+6	5.0	7.0	9.4
31+0 - 31+6	5.1	7.2	9.6
32+0 - 32+6	5.2	7.3	9.7
33+0 - 33+6	5.3	7.4	9.8
34+0 - 34+6	5.3	7.5	9.9
35+0 - 35+6	5.4	7.5	10.0
36+0 - 36+6	5.4	7.6	10.0
37+0 - 37+6	5.4	7.6	10.1
38+0 - 38+6	5.5	7.6	10.1
39+0 - 39+6	5.5	7.6	10.1

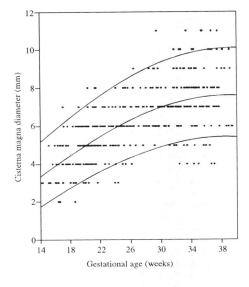

Table 8 Cerebral hemisphere diameter (mm).

Gestation	5th	median	95th
14+0 - 14+6	13	15	16
15+0 - 15+6	15	16	18
16+0 - 16+6	16	18	19
17+0 - 17+6	17	19	21
18+0 - 18+6	19	21	23
19+0 - 19+6	20	22	24
20+0 - 20+6	22	24	26
21+0 - 21+6	23	25	28
22+0 - 22+6	25	27	30
23+0 - 23+6	26	29	31
24+0 - 24+6	28	30	33
25+0 - 25+6	29	32	35
26+0 - 26+6	31	34	37
27+0 - 27+6	32	35	38
28+0 - 28+6	34	37	40
29+0 - 29+6	35	38	41
30+0 - 30+6	36	40	43
31+0 - 31+6	38	41	44
32+0 - 32+6	39	42	46
33+0 - 33+6	40	43	47
34+0 - 34+6	41	44	48
35+0 - 35+6	42	45	49
36+0 - 36+6	42	46	50
37+0 - 37+6	43	47	51
38+0 - 38+6	43	47	51
39+0 - 39+6	44	48	52

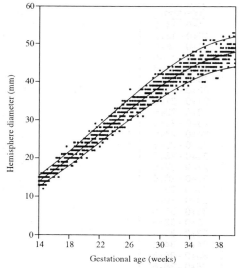

Table 9 Anterior cerebral ventricle diameter (mm).

Gestation	5th	median	95th
14+0 - 14+6	5.2	6.7	8.1
15+0 - 15+6	5.3	6.8	8.3
16+0 - 16+6	5.4	6.9	8.4
17+0 - 17+6	5.6	7.0	8.5
18+0 - 18+6	5.7	7.2	8.6
19+0 - 19+6	5.8	7.3	8.8
20+0 - 20+6	5.9	7.4	8.9
21+0 - 21+6	6.1	7.5	9.0
22+0 - 22+6	6.2	7.7	9.2
23+0 - 23+6	6.3	7.8	9.3
24+0 - 24+6	6.4	7.9	9.4
25+0 - 25+6	6.6	8.1	9.5
26+0 - 26+6	6.7	8.2	9.7
27+0 - 27+6	6.8	8.3	9.8
28+0 - 28+6	7.0	8.4	9.9
29+0 - 29+6	7.1	8.5	10.1
30+0 - 30+6	7.2	8.7	10.2
31+0 - 31+6	7.3	8.8	10.3
32+0 - 32+6	7.5	9.0	10.4
33+0 - 33+6	7.6	9.1	10.6
34+0 - 34+6	7.7	9.2	10.7
35+0 - 35+6	7.9	9.3	10.8
36+0 - 36+6	8.0	9.5	10.9
37+0 - 37+6	8.1	9.6	11.1
38+0 - 38+6	8.2	9.7	11.2
39+0 - 39+6	8.3	9.8	11.3

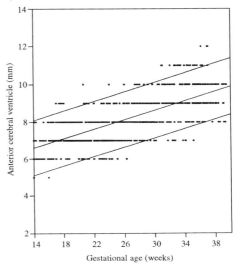

Table 10 Posterior cerebral ventricle diameter (mm).

Gestation	5th	median	95th
14+0 - 14+6	5.1	6.7	8.4
15+0 - 15+6	5.1	6.8	8.5
16+0 - 16+6	5.2	6.9	8.6
17+0 - 17+6	5.3	7.0	8.7
18+0 - 18+6	5.4	7.1	8.8
19+0 - 19+6	5.5	7.2	8.8
20+0 - 20+6	5.6	7.2	8.9
21+0 - 21+6	5.6	7.3	9.0
22+0 - 22+6	5.7	7.4	9.1
23+0 - 23+6	5.8	7.5	9.2
24+0 - 24+6	5.9	7.6	9.3
25+0 - 25+6	6.0	7.7	9.3
26+0 - 26+6	6.1	7.7	9.4
27+0 - 27+6	6.1	7.8	9.5
28+0 - 28+6	6.2	7.9	9.6
29+0 - 29+6	6.3	8.0	9.7
30+0 - 30+6	6.4	8.1	9.8
31+0 - 31+6	6.5	8.2	9.9
32+0 - 32+6	6.6	8.3	9.9
33+0 - 33+6	6.7	8.3	10.0
34+0 - 34+6	6.7	8.4	10.1
35+0 - 35+6	6.8	8.5	10.2
36+0 - 36+6	6.9	8.6	10.3
37+0 - 37+6	7.0	8.7	10.4
38+0 - 38+6	7.1	8.8	10.4
39+0 - 39+6	7.2	8.8	10.5

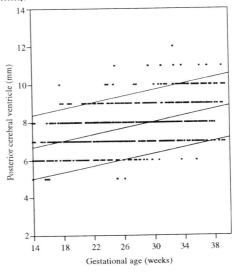

Table 11 Head to abdominal circumference ratio.

Gestation	5th	median	95th
14+0 - 14+6	1.12	1.23	1.33
15+0 - 15+6	1.11	1.22	1.32
16+0 - 16+6	1.10	1.21	1.31
17+0 - 17+6	1.09	1.20	1.30
18+0 - 18+6	1.09	1.19	1.29
19+0 - 19+6	1.08	1.18	1.29
20+0 - 20+6	1.07	1.17	1.28
21+0 - 21+6	1.06	1.16	1.27
22+0 - 22+6	1.05	1.15	1.26
23+0 - 23+6	1.04	1.14	1.25
24+0 - 24+6	1.03	1.13	1.24
25+0 - 25+6	1.02	1.12	1.23
26+0 - 26+6	1.01	1.11	1.22
27+0 - 27+6	1.00	1.10	1.21
28+0 - 28+6	0.99	1.09	1.20
29+0 - 29+6	0.98	1.08	1.19
30+0 - 30+6	0.97	1.08	1.18
31+0 - 31+6	0.96	1.07	1.17
32+0 - 32+6	0.95	1.06	1.16
33+0 - 33+6	0.94	1.05	1.15
34+0 - 34+6	0.93	1.04	1.14
35+0 - 35+6	0.92	1.03	1.13
36+0 - 36+6	0.91	1.02	1.12
37+0 - 37+6	0.90	1.01	1.11
38+0 - 38+6	0.89	1.00	1.10
39+0 - 39+6	0.88	0.99	1.09

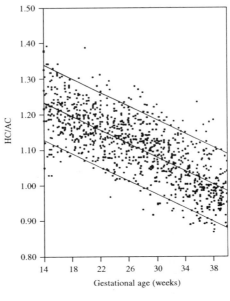

Table 12 Biparietal diameter to femur length ratio.

Gestation	5th	median	95th
14+0 - 14+6	1.70	1.87	2.06
15+0 - 15+6	1.62	1.78	1.95
16+0 - 16+6	1.55	1.70	1.87
17+0 - 17+6	1.49	1.64	1.80
18+0 - 18+6	1.45	1.59	1.74
19+0 - 19+6	1.41	1.54	1.69
20+0 - 20+6	1.37	1.51	1.66
21+0 - 21+6	1.35	1.48	1.62
22+0 - 22+6	1.33	1.46	1.60
23+0 - 23+6	1.31	1.44	1.58
24+0 - 24+6	1.30	1.43	1.57
25+0 - 25+6	1.29	1.42	1.56
26+0 - 26+6	1.29	1.41	1.55
27+0 - 27+6	1.28	1.41	1.54
28+0 - 28+6	1.28	1.40	1.54
29+0 - 29+6	1.28	1.40	1.54
30+0 - 30+6	1.28	1.40	1.54
31+0 - 31+6	1.27	1.40	1.53
32+0 - 32+6	1.27	1.39	1.53
33+0 - 33+6	1.27	1.39	1.53
34+0 - 34+6	1.26	1.37	1.52
35+0 - 35+6	1.25	1.36	1.51
36+0 - 36+6	1.24	1.34	1.49
37+0 - 37+6	1.22	1.32	1.47
38+0 - 38+6	1.20	1.30	1.45
39+0 - 39+6	1.18	1.28	1.42

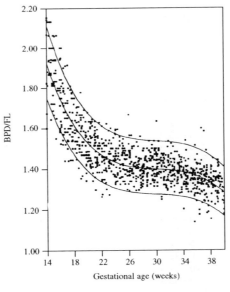

Table 13 Head circumference to femur length ratio.

Gestation	5th	median	95th
14+0 - 14+6	6.08	6.55	7.05
15+0 - 15+6	5.81	6.28	6.76
16+0 - 16+6	5.59	6.04	6.52
17+0 - 17+6	5.40	5.84	6.31
18+0 - 18+6	5.23	5.67	6.13
19+0 - 19+6	5.09	5.53	5.98
20+0 - 20+6	4.98	5.41	5.85
21+0 - 21+6	4.88	5.31	5.75
22+0 - 22+6	4.80	5.22	5.66
23+0 - 23+6	4.74	5.16	5.59
24+0 - 24+6	4.69	5.11	5.54
25+0 - 25+6	4.65	5.06	5.50
26+0 - 26+6	4.62	5.03	5.46
27+0 - 27+6	4.60	5.01	5.44
28+0 - 28+6	4.58	4.99	5.41
29+0 - 29+6	4.56	4.97	5.40
30+0 - 30+6	4.54	4.95	5.38
31+0 - 31+6	4.52	4.93	5.36
32+0 - 32+6	4.50	4.91	5.34
33+0 - 33+6	4.48	4.89	5.31
34+0 - 34+6	4.45	4.85	5.27
35+0 - 35+6	4.41	4.81	5.23
36+0 - 36+6	4.35	4.76	5.17
37+0 - 37+6	4.29	4.69	5.11
38+0 - 38+6	4.21	4.61	5.02
39+0 - 39+6	4.12	4.51	4.92

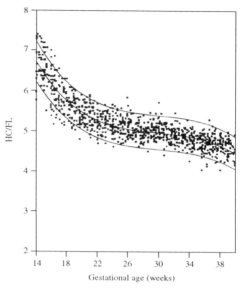

Table 14 Abdominal circumference to femur length ratio.

Gestation	5th	median	95th
14+0 - 14+6	4.82	5.40	6.04
15+0 - 15+6	4.64	5.19	5.81
16+0 - 16+6	4.49	5.03	5.62
17+0 - 17+6	4.37	4.89	5.47
18+0 - 18+6	4.27	4.78	5.34
19+0 - 19+6	4.19	4.69	5.24
20+0 - 20+6	4.13	4.62	5.16
21+0 - 21+6	4.08	4.56	5.10
22+0 - 22+6	4.05	4.53	5.06
23+0 - 23+6	4.03	4.50	5.04
24+0 - 24+6	4.02	4.49	5.02
25+0 - 25+6	4.02	4.49	5.02
26+0 - 26+6	4.02	4.50	5.03
27+0 - 27+6	4.04	4.51	5.05
28+0 - 28+6	4.05	4.53	5.07
29+0 - 29+6	4.08	4.56	5.10
30+0 - 30+6	4.10	4.58	5.13
31+0 - 31+6	4.12	4.61	5.16
32+0 - 32+6	4.15	4.64	5.19
33+0 - 33+6	4.17	4.66	5.22
34+0 - 34+6	4.19	4.69	5.24
35+0 - 35+6	4.20	4.70	5.26
36+0 - 36+6	4.21	4.71	5.27
37+0 - 37+6	4.21	4.70	5.27
38+0 - 38+6	4.20	4.68	5.26
39+0 - 39+6	4.18	4.66	5.23

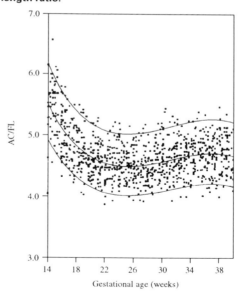

Table 15 Transverse cerebellar diameter to abdominal circumference ratio.

Gestation	5th	median	95th
14+0 - 14+6	0.139	0.157	0.175
15+0 - 15+6	0.135	0.153	0.171
16+0 - 16+6	0.131	0.149	0.167
17+0 - 17+6	0.127	0.145	0.163
18+0 - 18+6	0.125	0.142	0.160
19+0 - 19+6	0.122	0.140	0.158
20+0 - 20+6	0.120	0.138	0.156
21+0 - 21+6	0.118	0.136	0.154
22+0 - 22+6	0.117	0.135	0.153
23+0 - 23+6	0.116	0.134	0.152
24+0 - 24+6	0.115	0.133	0.151
25+0 - 25+6	0.115	0.133	0.151
26+0 - 26+6	0.115	0.132	0.150
27+0 - 27+6	0.114	0.132	0.150
28+0 - 28+6	0.114	0.132	0.150
29+0 - 29+6	0.115	0.132	0.150
30+0 - 30+6	0.115	0.133	0.151
31+0 - 31+6	0.115	0.133	0.151
32+0 - 32+6	0.115	0.133	0.151
33+0 - 33+6	0.115	0.133	0.151
34+0 - 34+6	0.115	0.133	0.151
35+0 - 35+6	0.115	0.133	0.151
36+0 - 36+6	0.115	0.133	0.151
37+0 - 37+6	0.115	0.133	0.151
38+0 - 38+6	0.114	0.132	0.150
39+0 - 39+6	0.113	0.131	0.149

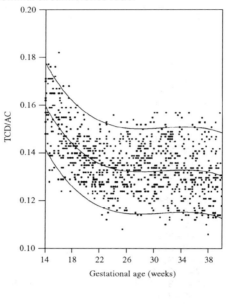

Table 16 Transverse cerebellar diameter to head circumference ratio.

Gestation	5th	median	95th
14+0 - 14+6	0.118	0.130	0.145
15+0 - 15+6	0.114	0.126	0.140
16+0 - 16+6	0.111	0.123	0.137
17+0 - 17+6	0.109	0.121	0.134
18+0 - 18+6	0.107	0.119	0.132
19+0 - 19+6	0.106	0.118	0.131
20+0 - 20+6	0.105	0.117	0.130
21+0 - 21+6	0.105	0.116	0.129
22+0 - 22+6	0.105	0.116	0.129
23+0 - 23+6	0.105	0.116	0.129
24+0 - 24+6	0.105	0.117	0.130
25+0 - 25+6	0.106	0.118	0.131
26+0 - 26+6	0.107	0.119	0.132
27+0 - 27+6	0.109	0.120	0.133
28+0 - 28+6	0.110	0.121	0.134
29+0 - 29+6	0.111	0.122	0.136
30+0 - 30+6	0.113	0.124	0.137
31+0 - 31+6	0.114	0.125	0.139
32+0 - 32+6	0.115	0.128	0.140
33+0 - 33+6	0.117	0.129	0.141
34+0 - 34+6	0.117	0.129	0.143
35+0 - 35+6	0.117	0.130	0.144
36+0 - 36+6	0.117	0.130	0.144
37+0 - 37+6	0.117	0.130	0.145
38+0 - 38+6	0.117	0.130	0.145
39+0 - 39+6	0.117	0.130	0.144

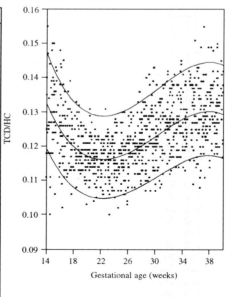

Table 17 Cerebral anterior ventricle to hemisphere diameter ratio.

Gestation	5th	median	95th
14+0 - 14+6	0.39	0.47	0.56
15+0 - 15+6	0.36	0.43	0.51
16+0 - 16+6	0.33	0.40	0.48
17+0 - 17+6	0.31	0.37	0.44
18+0 - 18+6	0.29	0.35	0.41
19+0 - 19+6	0.27	0.32	0.39
20+0 - 20+6	0.26	0.31	0.37
21+0 - 21+6	0.24	0.29	0.35
22+0 - 22+6	0.23	0.28	0.33
23+0 - 23+6	0.22	0.27	0.32
24+0 - 24+6	0.21	0.26	0.31
25+0 - 25+6	0.21	0.25	0.30
26+0 - 26+6	0.20	0.24	0.29
27+0 - 27+6	0.19	0.23	0.28
28+0 - 28+6	0.19	0.23	0.27
29+0 - 29+6	0.19	0.22	0.27
30+0 - 30+6	0.18	0.22	0.26
31+0 - 31+6	0.18	0.21	0.26
32+0 - 32+6	0.18	0.21	0.26
33+0 - 33+6	0.18	0.21	0.25
34+0 - 34+6	0.17	0.21	0.25
35+0 - 35+6	0.17	0.21	0.25
36+0 - 36+6	0.17	0.21	0.25
37+0 - 37+6	0.17	0.21	0.25
38+0 - 38+6	0.17	0.21	0.25
39+0 - 39+6	0.17	0.21	0.25

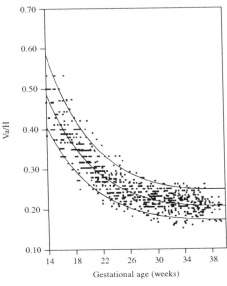

Table 18 Cerebral posterior ventricle to hemisphere diameter ratio.

Gestation	5th	median	95th
14+0 - 14+6	0.36	0.45	0.56
15+0 - 15+6	0.34	0.42	0.52
16+0 - 16+6	0.31	0.39	0.48
17+0 - 17+6	0.29	0.36	0.45
18+0 - 18+6	0.27	0.34	0.42
19+0 - 19+6	0.26	0.32	0.40
20+0 - 20+6	0.24	0.30	0.37
21+0 - 21+6	0.23	0.29	0.35
22+0 - 22+6	0.22	0.27	0.34
23+0 - 23+6	0.21	0.26	0.32
24+0 - 24+6	0.20	0.25	0.31
25+0 - 25+6	0.19	0.24	0.29
26+0 - 26+6	0.18	0.23	0.28
27+0 - 27+6	0.18	0.22	0.27
28+0 - 28+6	0.17	0.21	0.26
29+0 - 29+6	0.17	0.21	0.26
30+0 - 30+6	0.16	0.20	0.25
31+0 - 31+6	0.16	0.20	0.24
32+0 - 32+6	0.16	0.19	0.24
33+0 - 33+6	0.15	0.19	0.24
34+0 - 34+6	0.15	0.19	0.24
35+0 - 35+6	0.15	0.19	0.24
36+0 - 36+6	0.15	0.19	0.24
37+0 - 37+6	0.15	0.19	0.24
38+0 - 38+6	0.15	0.19	0.24
39+0 - 39+6	0.15	0.19	0.24

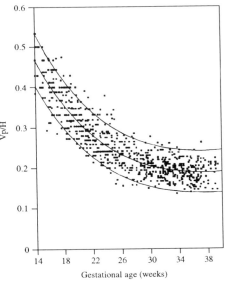

Table 19 Biparietal to occipitofrontal diameter ratio.

Gestation	5th	median	95th
14+0 - 14+6	0.75	0.80	0.86
15+0 - 15+6	0.74	0.80	0.86
16+0 - 16+6	0.74	0.80	0.86
17+0 - 17+6	0.74	0.79	0.85
18+0 - 18+6	0.74	0.79	0.85
19+0 - 19+6	0.73	0.79	0.85
20+0 - 20+6	0.73	0.79	0.85
21+0 - 21+6	0.73	0.79	0.85
22+0 - 22+6	0.73	0.79	0.85
23+0 - 23+6	0.73	0.79	0.85
24+0 - 24+6	0.73	0.79	0.85
25+0 - 25+6	0.73	0.79	0.85
26+0 - 26+6	0.73	0.79	0.85
27+0 - 27+6	0.73	0.79	0.85
28+0 - 28+6	0.74	0.79	0.85
29+0 - 29+6	0.74	0.79	0.85
30+0 - 30+6	0.74	0.79	0.85
31+0 - 31+6	0.74	0.80	0.86
32+0 - 32+6	0.74	0.80	0.86
33+0 - 33+6	0.75	0.80	0.86
34+0 - 34+6	0.75	0.81	0.87
35+0 - 35+6	0.75	0.81	0.87
36+0 - 36+6	0.76	0.82	0.88
37+0 - 37+6	0.76	0.82	0.88
38+0 - 38+6	0.77	0.83	0.89
39+0 - 39+6	0.77	0.83	0.90

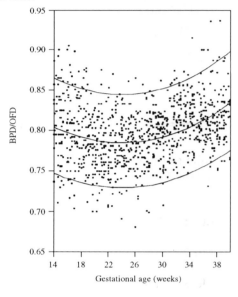

Appendix 2:
Estimated risks for chromosomal defects

Details of the methodology used to derive the estimated risks are discussed fully in Chapter 2.

Table 1 Trisomy 21

Table 2 Trisomy 18

Table 3 Trisomy 13

Table 4 Sex chromosome defects

Table 5 Choroid plexus cysts and trisomy 18

Table 6 Mild hydronephrosis and trisomy 21

Table 1 Trisomy 21: estimated risk (1/number given in the table) by maternal age and gestation.

Age (yrs)	Gestation (wks)									
	10	12	14	16	18	20	25	30	35	Birth
20	804	898	981	1053	1117	1175	1294	1388	1464	1527
21	793	887	968	1040	1103	1159	1277	1370	1445	1507
22	780	872	952	1022	1084	1140	1256	1347	1421	1482
23	762	852	930	999	1060	1114	1227	1317	1389	1448
24	740	827	903	969	1029	1081	1191	1278	1348	1406
25	712	795	868	933	989	1040	1146	1229	1297	1352
26	677	756	826	887	941	989	1090	1169	1233	1286
27	635	710	775	832	883	928	1022	1097	1157	1206
28	586	655	715	768	815	856	943	1012	1068	1113
29	531	593	648	695	738	776	855	917	967	1008
30	471	526	575	617	655	688	758	813	858	895
31	409	457	499	536	568	597	658	706	745	776
32	347	388	423	455	482	507	559	599	632	659
33	288	322	352	378	401	421	464	498	525	547
34	235	262	286	307	326	343	378	405	427	446
35	187	210	229	246	261	274	302	324	342	356
36	148	165	180	193	205	216	238	255	269	280
37	115	128	140	150	159	168	185	198	209	218
38	88	98	107	115	122	129	142	152	160	167
39	67	75	82	88	93	98	108	116	122	128
40	51	57	62	67	71	74	82	88	93	97
41	38	43	47	50	53	56	62	66	70	73
42	29	32	35	38	40	42	46	50	52	55
43	21	24	26	28	30	31	35	37	39	41
44	16	18	20	21	22	23	26	28	29	30

Table 2 Prevalence of trisomy 18 by maternal age and gestational age. Estimated risk (1/number given in the table).

Age (yrs)	Gestation (wks)									
	10	12	14	16	18	20	25	30	35	Birth
20	1993	2484	3015	3590	4215	4897	6909	9516	13028	18013
21	1968	2453	2976	3544	4160	4834	6820	9394	12860	17782
22	1934	2411	2925	3483	4090	4751	6704	9234	12641	17479
23	1891	2357	2860	3405	3998	4645	6553	9027	12357	17086
24	1835	2287	2776	3305	3880	4508	6361	8761	11994	16584
25	1765	2200	2670	3179	3732	4336	6118	8427	11536	15951
26	1679	2092	2539	3023	3549	4124	5819	8014	10972	15170
27	1575	1963	2382	2836	3330	3868	5458	7518	10292	14231
28	1453	1811	2198	2617	3073	3570	5037	6938	9498	13133
29	1316	1641	1991	2371	2783	3234	4562	6284	8603	11895
30	1168	1456	1766	2103	2469	2869	4048	5575	7633	10554
31	1014	1263	1533	1825	2143	2490	3513	4839	6625	9160
32	860	1072	1301	1549	1819	2114	2982	4107	5623	7775
33	715	891	1081	1287	1511	1755	2477	3412	4670	6458
34	582	725	880	1047	1230	1429	2016	2777	3802	5256
35	465	580	703	837	983	1142	1612	2220	3039	4202
36	366	456	553	659	774	899	1268	1747	2392	3307
37	284	354	430	512	601	698	985	1357	1858	2569
38	218	272	330	393	462	537	757	1043	1428	1974
39	167	208	252	300	352	409	577	795	1088	1505
40	126	157	191	227	267	310	437	602	824	1139
41	95	118	144	171	201	233	329	453	620	858
42	71	89	108	128	151	175	247	340	465	644
43	53	66	81	96	113	131	185	254	348	481
44	40	50	60	72	84	98	138	190	260	359

Table 3 Prevalence of trisomy 13 by maternal age and gestational age. Estimated risk (1/number given in the table).

Age (yrs)	Gestation (wks)									
	10	12	14	16	18	20	25	30	35	Birth
20	6347	7826	9389	11042	12795	14656	19854	26002	33387	42423
21	6266	7725	9268	10900	12630	14468	19599	25668	32958	41878
22	6159	7594	9110	10715	12415	14221	19265	25231	32397	41165
23	6021	7423	8906	10474	12137	13902	18832	24664	31669	40241
24	5844	7205	8644	10166	11780	13493	18279	23939	30738	39057
25	5621	6930	8314	9778	11330	12978	17581	23026	29565	37567
26	5345	6591	7907	9299	10776	12343	16721	21898	28118	35728
27	5014	6183	7417	8723	10108	11578	15685	20542	26376	33515
28	4628	5706	6845	8051	9329	10685	14475	18958	24342	30930
29	4191	5168	6200	7292	8449	9678	13111	17171	22048	28015
30	3719	4585	5501	6470	7496	8587	11632	15234	19561	24856
31	3228	3980	4774	5615	6507	7453	10096	13223	16978	21573
32	2740	3378	4052	4766	5523	6326	8570	11223	14411	18311
33	2275	2806	3366	3959	4587	5254	7118	9322	11969	15209
34	1852	2284	2740	3222	3734	4277	5794	7588	9743	12380
35	1481	1826	2190	2576	2985	3419	4631	6065	7788	9876
36	1165	1437	1724	2027	2349	2691	3645	4774	6129	7788
37	905	1116	1339	1575	1825	2090	2831	3708	4761	6050
38	696	858	1029	1210	1402	1606	2176	2850	3659	4650
39	530	654	784	922	1069	1224	1658	2172	2789	3544
40	401	495	594	698	809	927	1255	1644	2111	2683
41	302	373	447	526	609	698	946	1238	1590	2020
42	227	280	335	395	457	524	709	929	1193	1516
43	170	209	251	295	342	392	531	695	892	1134
44	127	156	187	220	255	292	396	519	666	846

Table 4 Sex chromosome defects: estimated risk (1/number in the table) by maternal age and gestation. For Turner syndrome the estimated risk is the same for all maternal ages. For 47,XXX, 47,XXY and 47,XYY, the risk is the same at all gestations.

Turner syndrome

Age (yrs)	Gestation (wks)									
	10	12	14	16	18	20	25	30	35	Birth
Any	538	1471	2083	2500	2857	3125	3571	3846	4000	4167

47,XXX

Age (yrs)	Same for all gestations
<35	2500
35-37	1667
38-40	1250
>40	1000

47,XXY

Age (yrs)	Same for all gestations
<35	1667
35-37	1250
38-40	1000
>40	833

47,XYY

Age (yrs)	Same for all gestations
<35	1667
35-37	2500
38-40	5000
>40	10000

Table 5 Choroid plexus cysts and trisomy 18. Estimated risk for trisomy 18 (1/number given in the table) in 20-week fetuses with isolated choroid plexus cysts, and in those with one and two or more additional abnormalities.

Age (yrs)	Total population	Choroid plexus cysts		Additional abnormalities		
		absent	present	0	1	≥2
20	4897	9793	98	3032	257	6
21	4834	9667	97	3001	254	6
22	4751	9501	95	2939	249	6
23	4645	9289	93	2876	244	6
24	4508	9015	90	2782	236	5
25	4336	8671	87	2689	228	5
26	4124	8247	82	2532	215	5
27	3868	7735	77	2376	202	5
28	3570	7139	71	2189	186	4
29	3234	6467	65	2001	170	4
30	2869	5737	57	1751	149	4
31	2490	4979	50	1532	130	3
32	2114	4227	42	1282	109	3
33	1755	3509	35	1064	91	3
34	1429	2857	29	876	75	2
35	1142	2283	23	689	59	2
36	899	1797	18	532	46	2
37	698	1395	14	407	35	2
38	537	1073	11	314	27	<2
39	409	817	8	220	19	<2
40	310	619	6	157	14	<2
41	233	465	5	126	12	<2
42	175	349	3	64	6	<2
43	131	261	3	64	6	<2
44	98	195	2	32	4	<2

Table 6 Mild hydronephrosis and trisomy 21. Estimated risk for trisomy 21 (1/number given in the table) in 20-week fetuses with isolated mild hydronephrosis and in those with one, two and three or more additional abnormalities.

Age (yrs)	Total population	Additional abnormalities			
		0	1	2	≥3
20	1175	735	80	26	22
21	1159	725	79	26	22
22	1140	713	77	26	21
23	1114	697	76	25	21
24	1081	676	73	24	20
25	1040	650	71	24	19
26	989	619	67	22	19
27	928	580	63	21	17
28	856	535	58	20	16
29	776	485	53	18	15
30	688	430	47	16	13
31	597	374	41	14	12
32	507	317	35	12	10
33	421	264	29	10	8
34	343	215	24	8	7
35	274	172	19	7	6
36	216	135	15	6	5
37	168	105	12	5	4
38	129	81	10	4	3
39	98	52	8	3	3
40	74	47	6	3	2
41	56	35	5	2	2
42	42	27	4	2	2
43	31	20	3	2	2
44	23	15	2	<2	<2

Index